CLINICAL EVALUATIONS OF SCHOOL-AGED CHILDREN

A Structured Approach to the Diagnosis of Child and Adolescent Mental Disorders

SUSAN K. SAMUELS / SUSANA SIKORSKY

Professional Resource Exchange, Inc.

Sarasota, FL

Paperback Edition ISBN: 0-943158-44-3
Library of Congress Catalog Card Number: 89-43664

The copy editor for this book was Janet Sailian, the managing editor was Debbie Fink, the graphics coordinator was Laurie Girsch, and the cover designer was Bill Tabler.

▌DEDICATION

To two special friends who have given us the support and encouragement through the best of times and the worst of times . . . to each other.

■ ACKNOWLEDGEMENT

Our gratitude to our professional colleagues in our local school districts and around the State of Connecticut for sharing their expertise, and graciously supporting this endeavor.

▌ TABLE OF CONTENTS

∎ PREFACE

Mental health professionals in schools need to communicate with a number of other professionals, such as psychiatrists and clinical psychologists involved in the assessment, diagnosis, and treatment of mental disorders in children and adolescents. Theoretical background, experience, knowledge, and practices among such professionals vary considerably, resulting in an array of differing terminology to describe a child's behavior and emotional status. *Clinical Evaluations of School-Aged Children: A Structured Approach to the Diagnosis of Child and Adolescent Mental Disorders* was created to bring about some uniformity in the behavioral considerations necessary for a given diagnosis.

Mental health professionals in schools must gather data, refine evaluations, respond to referral sources, prepare reports for clinical consultation, and interpret clinical findings to parents and school staff. One of the problems in communication between school personnel and outside professionals is the wide variation of terms used in the two different settings. Because most reports from clinicians include terms from the *Diagnostic and Statistical Manual of Mental Disorders: Third Edition - Revised* (*DSM-III-R*, 1987), knowledge of the specific criteria associated with each syndrome is necessary for school professionals as consultants in the school setting and liaison between schools and clinical practitioners. The reader should note that the syndromes described in the *DSM-III-R* are not the same as those described in earlier editions (*DSM-III*, 1980; *DSM-II*, 1968; *DSM-I*, 1952).

Clinical Evaluations of School-Aged Children: A Structured Approach to the Diagnosis of Child and Adolescent Mental Disorders focuses on the child and adolescent syndromes described in the *DSM-III-R*. Certain syndromes - such as Specific Developmental Disorders, including Developmental Arithmetic Disorder, Developmental Reading Disorder, and Developmental Expressive Writing Disorder - were excluded from this book because the criteria for determining abnormality in these areas vary considerably among states and school districts according to their particular diagnostic guidelines and policies. The diagnostic category of Mental Retardation has also been excluded from this book. In general, such diagnoses of primarily intellectual/academic deficiencies are routinely addressed by school personnel and do not necessarily warrant outside clinical consultation.

As the intent of this book is to clarify, differentiate, and cluster behaviors into well-defined syndromes, we have also excluded Undifferentiated Type diagnoses. Such classifications can be used by clinical practitioners when there is insufficient data or the data available does not meet the specific criteria for a given diagnosis (*DSM-III-R*).

In addition to the inclusion of all syndromes under the general category of Disorders First Evident in Infancy, Childhood, or Adolescence contained in the *DSM-III-R*, we have considered selected disorders whose onset may or may not occur during childhood, but whose manifestation is likely to concern school personnel.

Clinical Evaluations of School-Aged Children: A Structured Approach to the Diagnosis of Child and Adolescent Mental Disorders consists of three major inter-related components. The first is a Checklist of 15 symptoms whose presence or absence should routinely be considered as part of the diagnostic process. The second is a Comprehensive Summary of all characteristics for each disorder, including its associated features. The third is an Interview Form for use by mental health professionals when consulting with parents, teachers, and other school personnel.

The Checklist was designed to determine the presence or absence of such symptoms or behaviors as abnormal activity level, aggressiveness, anxiety, depression, inability to form or maintain social relationships, somatic complaints, hallucinations, delusions, language impairment, and impaired cognition. It also addresses such demographic variables as age of onset and duration of the syndrome. This Checklist will not, by itself, provide a comprehensive understanding of each disorder, but it may serve as an initial screening to consider or exclude any one diagnosis.

A Comprehensive Summary of all characteristics included in each disorder follows the Checklist. This section is vital in understanding a given syndrome. It includes all pertinent and associated features, and summarizes all the components that need to be considered to differentiate among a variety of syndromes. To insure clarity, each description is based on the corresponding text found in the *DSM-III-R*. It is presented in objective terms allowing close comparison between the behaviors or symptoms of the referred child and those characteristics found in the Comprehensive Summary.

The Interview Form was developed to facilitate gathering information from different sources. It was specifically designed to follow diagnostic considerations and other environmental and familial factors outlined in the *DSM-III-R*. It is an essential component, since it allows for an objective description of behaviors or symptoms and an expanded view of the child in a variety of settings.

Case histories have been included to illustrate the capacity of *Clinical Evaluations of School-Aged Children: A Structured Approach to the Diagnosis of Child and Adolescent Mental Disorders* to confirm a given diagnosis, and to suggest areas that could be productively explored by those working with the child.

The reader is cautioned that many of the categories described in the *DSM-III-R* have questionable inter-rater reliability. Nonetheless, it is today the most widely used reference manual among clinical practitioners. This book has been developed primarily to assist mental health professionals in the organization and preparation of data. It does not replace the *DSM-III-R* or the appropriate use of psychological testing, nor was it designed to provide a final clinical diagnosis.

However, we believe that the flexible design of *Clinical Evaluations of School-Aged Children: A Structured Approach to the Diagnosis of Child and Adolescent Mental Disorders* will enable mental health professionals to organize and expand on available information from a variety of perspectives. It provides structure and direction in gathering data, following the initial referral. This should lead to clearer and more precise communication, either to the clinical practitioner or to parents and others in the school setting.

REFERENCES

American Psychiatric Association. (1952). *Diagnostic and Statistical Manual of Mental Disorders* (1st ed.). Washington, DC: Author.

American Psychiatric Association. (1968). *Diagnostic and Statistical Manual of Mental Disorders* (2nd ed.). Washington, DC: Author.

American Psychiatric Association. (1980). *Diagnostic and Statistical Manual of Mental Disorders* (3rd ed.). Washington, DC: Author.

American Psychiatric Association. (1987). *Diagnostic and Statistical Manual of Mental Disorders* (3rd ed. rev.). Washington, DC: Author.

DISRUPTIVE BEHAVIOR DISORDERS

INTRODUCTION

Disruptive Behavior Disorders include Attention Deficit Hyperactivity Disorder, Conduct Disorders, and Oppositional Defiant Disorder. All share externalizing symptoms associated with social disruption. They tend to be more distressing to others than to the identified individuals themselves.

ATTENTION DEFICIT
HYPERACTIVITY DISORDER

The *DSM-III* previously considered three subtypes of this disorder: Attention Deficit Disorder with Hyperactivity, Attention Deficit Disorder without Hyperactivity, and a Residual type.

In the present diagnostic schema, Attention Deficit Hyperactivity Disorder (ADHD) is characterized by developmentally inappropriate inattention, impulsivity, and hyperactivity. All three symptoms are usually present, but they may vary in degree. For example, in preschool children, the most prominent feature may be gross motor overactivity, such as excessive climbing and running. In adolescents, the most salient feature may be impulsiveness in social situations, such as an abrupt decision to go joyriding instead of attending a planned event.

Hyperactivity is often characterized by restlessness, fidgeting, excessive running, and inability to sit still for an age-appropriate length of time. The lack of goal-directed, organized motor activity differentiates this disorder from ordinary overactivity. The level of hyperactivity varies with the child, his or her age, and the structural organization of the environment. For example, the child's behavior may seem appropriate in a new, one-to-one, or small-group situation, but it may become disorganized in a large-group setting. Different degrees of hyperactivity may be seen in school during such times as lunch, independent work periods, recess, or in teacher-directed lessons.

3

At home, these children may be involved in excessively noisy activities, frequently shifting from one to another. They often interrupt or intrude in the family routine, and have trouble following through with verbal requests. They tend to be accident-prone because of carelessness.

Inattention in school may be manifested by poor listening skills, and inability to complete tasks or organize work. Because these children are unable to sustain attention, they tend to be careless in their school work. Impulsivity may be noted by their difficulty in taking turns, acting before thinking, and calling out frequently. Children with this disorder may engage in potentially harmful activities because they do not think through the consequences of their actions. Such disruptions do not necessarily imply malicious intent.

In both home and school, these children have difficulty following social and game rules. Their behavior may be characterized by excessive talking, inability to take turns, and disruptions in social conventions. The behaviors associated with hyperactivity, inattention, and impulsivity in children with this syndrome usually necessitate frequent adult supervision.

Among the associated features of this disorder are low self-esteem and difficulty with interpersonal relationships. Attitudes and behaviors may include mood swings, low frustration tolerance, temper tantrums, bullying, bossiness, negativism, stubbornness, obstinacy, and poor responses to authority. Children with Attention Deficit Hyperactivity Disorder are at risk for developing Oppositional Defiant Disorder and Conduct Disorders, and are more likely to experience school failure.

(Consult Checklist on page 5.)

ATTENTION DEFICIT HYPERACTIVITY DISORDER INTERVIEW FORM

The following questions associated with ADHD are listed in descending order of discriminating power.

1. Does the child fidget excessively (in younger children, squirming in seat; in adolescents, feelings of restlessness)?

CHECKLIST

ATTENTION DEFICIT
HYPERACTIVITY DISORDER

Major Symptoms:

Key

+	Inattention
+	Impulsivity
+	Abnormal Activity Level
-	Aggressiveness
-	Violation of Rules
-	Isolation/Withdrawal/Avoidance
*	Inability to Form/Maintain Relationships
-	Disturbances of Affect or Mood
-	Anxiety
-	Depression
-	Delusions/Hallucinations
-	Somatic Complaints
-	Oddities of Behavior
-	Language Impairment
-	Impaired Cognition

Key:
+ Presence
- Absence
* Associated Feature

Demographic Variables:

Age of Onset: Before age 7.
Duration: At least 6 months.

5

2. Does the child have difficulty remaining seated when required to do so?
3. Is the child easily distracted by surrounding noises or people?
4. Does the child have difficulty waiting his or her turn in games or group situations?
5. Does the child blurt out answers to questions before they have been completed?
6. Does the child often fail to finish things he or she starts?
7. Is the child able to sustain attention in schoolwork or play activities?
8. Does the child often and unintentionally shift from one uncompleted activity to another?
9. Does the child have difficulty playing quietly?
10. Does the child often talk incessantly as though his or her mind is going a mile a minute?
11. Does the child often interrupt or encroach on others?
12. Does he or she often appear not to listen?
13. Does the child have difficulty organizing himself or herself; for example, losing pencils, books, or toys, in school or at home?
14. Does the child engage in physically harmful behaviors without considering their consequences? Describe.
15. At what age and for how long have these behaviors been noticed?
16. Are those reporting on the child aware of age-appropriate norms and behavioral expectations?
17. What are the child's responses to authority's attempts at discipline?
18. What are the child's attitudes and behaviors towards peers?
19. Does the child become easily frustrated and feel as though he or she cannot accomplish what is expected?
20. Have nonlocalized "soft" neurological signs, motor-perceptual dysfunction, and/or EEG abnormalities been reported?

Criteria for Severity: The *DSM-III-R* bases the severity of ADHD on the effect that symptoms have on school and social functioning. It ranges from mild to moderate to severe. For example, mild ADHD would indicate minimum or no effect on functioning, while severe

ADHD means more than the minimal number of symptoms necessary for diagnosis with a sustained effect on home, school, and social functioning.

The authors of this book strongly caution practitioners in their assessment of this disorder, since adults may vary in their observations, interactions, and tolerance for children's externalizing behaviors.

ATTENTION DEFICIT HYPERACTIVITY DISORDER
CASE SUMMARY - Andy, C.A., 4-10

Reason for Referral: Andy, a preschool child, was referred for evaluation because of concerns with his behavior. He was extremely active, distractible, and oppositional. Because of his behavior, Andy was dismissed from a town's nursery school program. Although active most of the time, Andy could reportedly sit for as long as 30 minutes, either watching television or playing with his Legos.

Consultant's Report: For the first 15 minutes of the session, Andy constantly tried to get out of his seat. The psychologist had to hold Andy's chair next to the table, but even with those restraints, he was out of the seat several times.

The most noticeable factor influencing Andy's intelligence testing scores was his inability to concentrate and respond to verbal directions. When asked a question, his answers were barely related. For instance, when shown a thumb and asked to name it, he answered "mouth"; when asked what lives in water, he answered "water in the sink, clean the dishes." It was unclear whether Andy misunderstood the question, was not able to comprehend the words, or was too distracted to hear the complete question.

In summary, Andy was an active 4-year-old who demonstrated distractible behaviors. Although he was seen for three sessions, Andy was unable to attend long enough to allow a valid estimate of his intellectual potential. The major recommendation was for Andy's parents to address the issue of behavior management.

Psychiatric Consultation: Andy has just been removed from a local nursery school. Both his teacher and parents feel that Andy will not be able to function in a regular kindergarten. He obeys the teacher but is very

7

active and distractible. His attention span is about 1-1/2 minutes. He talks endlessly, jumping from one subject to another, and it is difficult to follow what he is saying. Andy learns better on a one-to-one basis, but he can't seem to grasp some things. He is significantly low on readiness skills and may cry if he can't get his way. Andy is bossy and manipulative with peers. They seem to tolerate him and play alongside him, but real friendship is questionable.

Andy's activity level is consistently very high. He frequently shifts his interest and attention. His performance on tests of fine motor coordination is poor. There is a strong indication that Andy is suffering from an Attention Deficit Hyperactivity Disorder with severe impairment, attested to by failure in school, inability to be managed at home, and poor peer relationships. I recommend that he be re-evaluated just before the beginning of school by his pediatrician or child psychiatrist. Stimulant medication may be necessary, and some behaviorally oriented psychotherapy will almost certainly be needed. In school, I recommend a highly structured, self-contained classroom.

AUTHORS' COMMENTS

Andy manifests at least 9 of the 14 symptoms required for diagnosis of Attention Deficit Hyperactivity Disorder according to the *DSM-III-R*. For example, he is unable to follow directions, is highly distractible, and is unable to concentrate in schoolwork. Andy's excessive activity levels further illustrate the presence of this disorder.

Andy also displays several additional features associated with ADHD, such as bossiness, oppositional tendencies, manipulative behaviors, and poor school performance, as evidenced by his dismissal from nursery school and low readiness skills. His deficient performance on many perceptual-motor tasks is also characteristic of some children with ADHD, suggesting the possibility of neurological involvement.

CONDUCT DISORDERS

The major characteristic of these disorders is a long-term, recurrent pattern of behaviors that violate the basic rights of others or major age-appropriate societal rules and norms. The seriousness of such behaviors differentiates this group of disorders from the common mischief and antics of children and adolescents.

Four major subtypes of Conduct Disorder were considered in the *DSM-III*: Undersocialized Aggressive, Undersocialized Nonaggressive, Socialized Aggressive, and Socialized Nonaggressive. The *DSM-III-R* includes only three types of Conduct Disorder: Solitary Aggressive Type (roughly corresponding to the Undersocialized Aggressive), Group Type (roughly corresponding to the Socialized Nonaggressive), and Undifferentiated Type.

Predisposition to all three subtypes of this disorder may include Attention Deficit Hyperactivity Disorder, poor parenting skills, absence of parental figures, rejection or instability in the home environment, and associations with delinquent groups. All three subtypes show a long-term pattern of behavioral difficulties at home and in the community. Precocious sexual activity, drug abuse (drinking and smoking) at an early age, vexing, and recklessness are often present. Low self-esteem is usually masked by an air of toughness. In school, children with Conduct Disorder tend to be underachievers, inattentive, and often have low verbal skills and reading difficulties. At home and in school, these children show irritability, temper tantrums, and poor frustration tolerance. Symptoms of anxiety and depression may be common.

Such children usually manipulate others for advantage and show no guilt or remorse for their actions. They do not express concern for the feelings, wishes, or wellbeing of their peers, and seem inconsiderate and self-centered. When caught, they appear unable to accept responsibility for their behaviors, tending to inform on and blame others.

SOLITARY AGGRESSIVE TYPE

This disorder is manifested by aggressiveness towards people and property. Aggressiveness towards others involves a prolonged pattern of physical violence and/or confrontational behaviors. Often such individuals present a history of vandalism, rape, fire-setting, mugging, assault, extortion, or armed robbery. Frequently, this aggressive pattern is directed towards others outside of the home. However, in some instances, the parents of the individual may be the victims. In this type of Conduct Disorder, aggressiveness is initiated by the individual, not as part of a gang or group.

GROUP TYPE

This disorder is manifested by a long-term pattern involving violations of age-appropriate rules and possible aggressiveness towards people and property, but with some evidence of social attachments. Some indications of socialized behaviors may include sustained peer-group friendships, concern for the welfare of companions, and apparent feelings of guilt and remorse even when not directly challenged. These individuals are likely to refrain from blaming others and often will extend themselves to peers even when there is no immediate gain. However, they do not apply the same appropriate social skills outside their tight circle of friends. With strangers or with those to whom they are not affectively attached, they tend to show more manipulative and callous behavior, with no evidence of guilt or remorse for their actions.

UNDIFFERENTIATED TYPE

This type of disorder includes a mixture of symptoms found in both the Solitary Aggressive and Group types.

(Consult Checklists on pages 11 and 12.)

CONDUCT DISORDERS
INTERVIEW FORM

The following questions are listed in descending order of discriminating power.

1. Has the child been involved in stealing surreptitiously without confronting the victim?
2. Has he or she repeatedly run away from home (at least twice, or once without returning)?
3. Is he or she a persistent and serious liar?
4. Has he or she deliberately engaged in fire-setting?
5. Is he or she persistently truant from school?
6. Does he or she engage in breaking and entering?
7. Does he or she exhibit evidence of physical violence against persons or property, such as vandalism?

CHECKLIST

CONDUCT DISORDER, SOLITARY AGGRESSIVE TYPE

Major Symptoms:

Key

*	Inattention
-	Impulsivity
-	Abnormal Activity Level
+	Aggressiveness
+	Violation of Rules
+	Isolation/Withdrawal/Avoidance
+	Inability to Form/Maintain Relationships
-	Disturbances of Affect or Mood
*	Anxiety
*	Depression
-	Delusions/Hallucinations
-	Somatic Complaints
-	Oddities of Behavior
-	Language Impairment
*	Impaired Cognition

Key:
+ Presence
- Absence
* Associated Feature

Demographic Variables:

Age of Onset: Prepubertal.
Duration: At least 6 months.

11

CHECKLIST

CONDUCT DISORDER, GROUP TYPE

Major Symptoms:

Key

*	Inattention
-	Impulsivity
-	Abnormal Activity Level
+	Aggressiveness
+	Violation of Rules
-	Isolation/Withdrawal/Avoidance
-	Inability to Form/Maintain Relationships
-	Disturbances of Affect or Mood
*	Anxiety
*	Depression
-	Delusions/Hallucinations
-	Somatic Complaints
-	Oddities of Behavior
-	Language Impairment
*	Impaired Cognition

Key
+ Presence
- Absence
* Associated Feature

Demographic Variables:

Age of Onset: Pubertal or Postpubertal.
Duration: At least 6 months.

12

8. Does he or she engage in physical cruelty towards animals?
9. Has he or she forced someone into sexual activity?
10. Has he or she used a weapon more than once while fighting?
11. Does he or she often initiate physical fights?
12. Has he or she committed thefts involving confrontation with the victim, such as extortion, purse snatching, or armed robbery?
13. Has he or she been physically cruel to people?
14. For how long has this behavior pattern been evident?
15. Is he or she able to express guilt or remorse when appropriate?
16. Does he or she generally avoid blaming or reporting on companions?
17. Is he or she generally concerned for the welfare of others?
18. What is his or her achievement in school compared to his or her learning potential?
19. For how long can he or she attend or concentrate on school related tasks?
20. When antisocial acts are committed, is he or she involved alone or as part of a group or gang?

Note: Question number 20 will help differentiate between Solitary Aggressive and Group subtypes.

Criteria for Severity: Criteria to determine the severity of the disorder (Mild, Moderate, and Severe) is considered in the *DSM-III-R*. A mild disorder is diagnosed when few conduct problems are present and cause only minor harm to others. A severe disorder is diagnosed when the number of behaviors exceeds the minimum criteria for diagnosis or when such behaviors cause serious harm to others.

CONDUCT DISORDER, SOLITARY AGGRESSIVE TYPE
CASE SUMMARY - Luis, C.A., 15-4

Referral Reason: Luis frequently does not take responsibility for getting himself to school, and engages in a number of problematic behaviors at school - including temper outbursts, refusal to perform tasks, wide mood swings, and problems with his interpersonal relationships.

13

He does not appear to take responsibility for his actions and has no goal orientation. He is reportedly a self-centered youngster, whose academic performance has often been good; on at least one occasion he made the honor role. He was referred to Juvenile Court for malicious mischief and reportedly has been quite aggressive towards his peers.

Background Information: On the psychological evaluation, Luis' intellectual performance on the WISC-R placed him in the bright average range of intellectual functioning. There was a large disparity between his verbal and performance scores, resulting in his Verbal IQ being in the Average range, whereas his Performance IQ was in the Superior group. He apparently at one time was engaged in fecal soiling. Luis does have a history of seizures for which he has taken Dilantin for some period of time. A referral to Protective Services was made 2 years ago when Luis was reported as beyond control and because he had engaged in runaway behaviors.

Mother reports that while she is away at work, Luis brings acquaintances home. Since they smoke a great deal, she is fearful that he will start a fire in their house. They use "dirty language," smoke marijuana, and drink. At times Luis stays out all night. He too, uses marijuana and drinks alcohol. Her husband, from whom she is currently separated, and Luis, are often in conflict with each other. In contrast to Luis, father gets along well with his other two sons.

Luis arrived at the interview accompanied by the school psychologist. He entered the interview room readily and without noticeable signs of anxiety. Discussing his schoolwork, Luis commented that it was a "normal routine." It was apparent that he was quite evasive and wished to avoid disclosure of school-related problems. Probed for this school year's grades, Luis stated that he got four F's. The evaluator found it necessary to extract information piece by piece. Luis disclosed that he was in a special program. Further, he was suspended frequently for such things as breaking a school window, fighting, and disruptive behavior.

Diagnosis: Conduct Disorder, Solitary Aggressive Type, Severe.

Recommendations:

1. Placement in a residential center of a highly structured type with a policy of firm limit-setting. It is advisable that his parents become involved in family-oriented psychotherapy while Luis resides in the placement center.
2. Since Luis refuses to take responsibility for his actions, it is important that limit-setting within the confines of the classroom be clear and definite with specific consequences for his negative behaviors.

AUTHORS' COMMENTS

In the Solitary Aggressive Type, the child presents a long-term pattern of physical aggressiveness towards others as well as difficulties with interpersonal relationships. Luis is seen as a self-centered youngster, who is out of control at home and in school, as evidenced by his truancy, frequent suspensions for fighting, attempts to run away, smoking marijuana, drinking, and breaking and entering. Although he associates with others, these relationships appear to be superficial at best and center around illegal activities. However, most disruptive behaviors seem to be initiated by Luis and carried out on his own.

In addition, Luis' encopresis until age 11 may be viewed as further evidence of emotional difficulties. Because of his behavior, he has been unable to achieve in school, given his good intellectual potential. The severity of Luis' antisocial behaviors warranted removal from the mainstream and placement in an institutional setting.

CONDUCT DISORDER, GROUP TYPE
CASE SUMMARY - Charles, C.A., 13-0

Reason for Referral: Charles, chronologically a 7th grader, has experienced significant difficulties this year and last year at his school in work completion, interpersonal relationships, and appropriate school behavior. He is often absent and exhibits little concern about completing work. He takes little responsibility for his actions and is very creative in his use of excuses, sometimes becoming oppositional and disrespectful towards adults. Bus behavior is a problem. Recently, he punched another child in the face and was suspended for 4 days.

He has received direct service in the Learning Center due to a learning disability. Charles currently functions below customary 6th grade academic expectations. He has spotty skill development, with some mastery at the 4th, 5th, and 6th grade levels.

Since kindergarten, Charles has experienced academic difficulties. A proposed 3rd grade retention, opposed by his mother, resulted in evaluation and diagnosis of Learning Disabilities. School reports reflect a history of task avoidance, lack of motivation in the school setting, and a defiant attitude.

Charles lives with his mother and two older brothers. Mother currently works two jobs. His parents are divorced and his father has maintained some contact with the children over the years.

Findings and Recommendations: Charles was not spontaneous in conversation. He had many reasons for his difficulty in school, such as, "Don't understand directions," "sloppy," and "lazy"; he also had excuses for not doing homework and for being late.

Charles told the examiner about shooting cows in the rear with his b.b. gun, commenting that he likes to see them jump and make noise. He responded to the formal testing rather passively, often leaning on his elbow and delivering his responses in a flat tone.

Projective testing and observation of behavior suggest that Charles has adjustment difficulties. He reveals himself to be an immature, angry, insecure child who is experiencing considerable inner anxiety, a child who is still at odds with authority, and whose handling of drives is unsuccessful.

Evident throughout the testing were Charles' oppositional tendencies. Significant hostility and Charles' hypercritical attitude towards others obstruct empathetic relations and interfere with an appropriately developing value system. Charles' emotional responses also tend to be impulsive and infantile. He may respond superficially, more in terms of what he feels is demanded by the situation than to its reality.

16

Charles' high number of detailed responses to the Rorschach cards suggested an obsessive-compulsive personality, one which may over-react rather than respond appropriately to the demands of the stimuli. The stories that Charles related in response to the TAT cards contained people who were passive, unmotivated, and unaccepting of responsibility.

Psychiatric Consultant: Charles came to the interview willingly. He related rather coldly and callously at first, but was able to respond more appropriately when effectively confronted. His affect was appropriate to his mood.

Charles' mentation was clear in most areas, with the outstanding exception of his thoughts about authority. He attempted to use a variety of verbal manipulations when questioned about this issue. When these failed, he finally and reluctantly admitted that he fails to acknowledge the authority of school personnel when he feels like it.

I feel that Charles is experiencing a Conduct Disorder Group Type, Mild. If this pattern were to continue, it could lead to the development of an Antisocial Personality Disorder. I recommend a high degree of structure in the school environment. He seems to confuse authority with freedom of thought. It is important that he learn to distinguish between those two factors. To that end, Charles' mother agreed to intercede on behalf of school personnel whenever the boy acts rebelliously in school.

AUTHORS' COMMENTS

Charles' behavior indicates aggressiveness towards others, some instances of assault to children, cruelty to animals, low self-esteem, and difficulties with school-related tasks. His achievement level is below his intellectual potential, and he has been receiving services in the Learning Disabilities classroom. Background history reveals inconsistent limit-setting and intermittent presence of parental figures.

These behavioral patterns would constitute a Conduct Disorder. However, the Group Type component cannot be easily determined by this case, since neither the school psychologist nor the consultant psychiatrist explored Charles' quality of social relationships, or his ability to maintain peer friendships. At present, Charles' behaviors meet the minimum criteria for diagnosis of Conduct Disorder, warranting a determination of mild degree.

OPPOSITIONAL DEFIANT DISORDER

This disorder is characterized by a persistent antagonistic attitude, especially towards authority figures such as parents and teachers, after the developmental age when oppositional behaviors are frequent (18-36 months of age). Behaviors such as negativism, swearing, provocativeness, disobedience, stubbornness, argumentativeness, procrastination, and passive resistance are common, even when they are obviously against the self-interest and well-being of the child or adolescent.

Most often the individual sees others as the cause of his or her difficulties; he or she is unable to assume responsibility and views others as demanding and essentially unreasonable. Frequent behaviors include violations of minor rules, opposition to any suggestions, refusal to follow directions, and inability to refrain from carrying out an act which has been specifically forbidden. School and family difficulties are commonly associated with this disorder. Social relationships may be affected because of the hostile, oppositional attitude exhibited by these children, even when engaged in pleasurable peer activities. Depending upon the child's age, there may be use of illegal substances, such as tobacco, alcohol, and cannabis.

This pattern of confrontation is generally more upsetting and disruptive to the adults than to the child. Oppositional behaviors are more commonly manifested with people who are familiar to the child. During formal evaluation in a clinical setting, these behaviors may not be evident. Therefore, it may be necessary to gather specific data from sources familiar with the child rather than base a diagnosis solely on the clinical assessment.

All the features of the Oppositional Defiant Disorder may be present in the Conduct Disorders. The latter involve violations of major rules and basic rights of others. For this reason, diagnosis of Conduct Disorder would preempt a diagnosis of Oppositional Defiant Disorder. In some cases, Attention Deficit Hyperactivity Disorder may also be present, warranting a separate diagnosis.

CHECKLIST

OPPOSITIONAL DEFIANT DISORDER

Major Symptoms:

Key

-	Inattention
-	Impulsivity
-	Abnormal Activity Level
+	Aggressiveness
+	Violation of Rules
-	Isolation/Withdrawal/Avoidance
*	Inability to Form/Maintain Relationships
-	Disturbances of Affect or Mood
-	Anxiety
-	Depression
-	Delusions/Hallucinations
-	Somatic Complaints
-	Oddities of Behavior
-	Language Impairment
-	Impaired Cognition

Key

+ Presence

- Absence

* Associated Feature

Demographic Variables:

Age of Onset: After age 3, before age 18.
Duration: At least 6 months.

19

OPPOSITIONAL DEFIANT DISORDER INTERVIEW FORM

The following questions associated with Oppositional Defiant Disorder are listed in descending order of discriminating power.

1. Does the child often lose his or her temper?
2. Does he or she often argue with adults?
3. Does he or she often blatantly refuse to comply with adult requests or rules?
4. Does he or she purposely do things to annoy others?
5. Does he or she usually blame others for his or her difficulties?
6. Does he or she appear touchy and easily annoyed by others?
7. Does he or she often appear angry and resentful?
8. Is he or she reported to be vindictive or spiteful?
9. Does he or she often swear and use obscenities?
10. Do such behaviors persist even when they interfere with the child's receiving positive reinforcement, such as concrete rewards, adult attention, and good grades?
11. Do these behaviors extend to the violation of major rules and the basic rights of others; for example, theft, vandalism, physical aggression, persistent truancy, and drug abuse?
12. To what extent is the family and/or school affected by the child's behavior?
13. To what extent are the child's peer relationships affected by his or her oppositional attitude?
14. For how long has this pattern of behavior been present?

Criteria for Severity: A mild degree is diagnosed when few symptoms are present and only cause minor impairment in school and social functioning. A severe degree is diagnosed when symptoms exceed the minimum criteria for diagnosis and when there is significant impairment at home and school, and with other adults and peers.

OPPOSITIONAL DEFIANT DISORDER
CASE SUMMARY - Abe, C.A., 14-0

Reason for Referral: Abe was referred for evaluation because of behavior problems in school and at home, and poor relationships with family members. He is reported to be an angry, argumentative youngster, often refusing to comply with simple parental requests. At school, Abe teases other children, and when confronted about his behavior, he quickly blames his peers. His use of obscene language has warranted removal from class and several suspensions.

Consultant's Report: Abe demonstrates considerable immaturity. There is out-of-control behavior of an aggressive and oppositional nature, and a great deal of resentment towards his younger brother. This resentment was recently displayed by two incidents; one in which he threw sand into his brother's eyes, and another in which he threw ammonia into his brother's eyes. Both of these were treated as accidents by mother, suggesting denial and poor ability on her part to generate control over his behavior.

Abe also has a tendency to be extremely manipulative and to make excuses for his behaviors, indicating that they are caused by other people. He has an extremely low frustration tolerance and is virtually unwilling to do anything that appears work-like in school.

In this instance, the diagnosis is Oppositional Defiant Disorder, Moderate.

Recommendations:

1. Without intervention, Abe is seriously at risk for developing a Conduct Disorder. Therefore, it is recommended that Abe see a counselor with his mother to establish behavioral controls, and to support his mother through the resentment and acting-out behavior that is likely to occur during the establishment of these behavioral controls.
2. The school should consider placement in a special class for behaviorally disordered children.

AUTHORS' COMMENTS

Abe's oppositional behaviors, as characterized by his resistance to schoolwork and provocative attitude at school and towards his family members, are two patterns found in Oppositional Defiant Disorder. In addition, Abe frequently confronts his mother to the point where she can no longer control him.

Abe's aggressive acts are potentially dangerous to his brother, and thus could be construed as the beginning stages of a Conduct Disorder.

It is important to determine what Abe's response to behavioral modification techniques has been thus far, because very often these children do not respond well to positive reinforcement.

Another common feature of children with this disorder is poor peer relationships because of a pervasive antagonistic attitude, even when engaged in play activities. Therefore, the evaluation should have included some specificity regarding Abe's interactions with peers.

ADDITIONAL READINGS FOR
DISRUPTIVE BEHAVIOR DISORDERS

Achenbach, T. M. (1982). *Developmental Psychopathology* (2nd ed.). New York: John Wiley.

Barkley, R. A. (1981). *Hyperactive Children.* New York: Guilford.

Barkley, R. A. (1987). *Defiant Children.* New York: Guilford.

Kazdin, A. E. (1987). *Conduct Disorders in Childhood and Adolescence.* Beverly Hills: Sage.

Martin, H. (1987). *Conduct Disorders of Childhood and Adolescence: A Social Learning Perspective.* New York: John Wiley.

Rutter, M., & Giller, H. (1984). *Juvenile Delinquency.* New York: Guilford.

ANXIETY DISORDERS

AVOIDANT DISORDER OF
CHILDHOOD OR ADOLESCENCE

Anxiety in this disorder is manifested by excessive shrinking from social situations occurring after the developmental age when "stranger anxiety" is common (usually 2-1/2 years of age). Social avoidance may be demonstrated by timidity, embarrassment, inhibition of communication skills, and lack of initiative with others. Excessive avoidant behavior may result in poor social functioning, particularly with peers.

Children with this disorder most often have warm family relationships, are eager for affection, and desire participation in social activities. However, once confronted with demands for contact with others outside their family circle, they become inarticulate, tearful, and overly dependent upon family members. These children are frequently described as lacking self-confidence and assertiveness. In adolescence, inhibition of interest in psychosexual activity may be found. Socially reticent children may be slow to warm up to an unfamiliar situation, but with time they are able to interact appropriately with others. Avoidant children, however, continue a pattern of social shrinking and suffer impairment in peer relationships.

Children with this disorder may also show symptoms of other anxiety disorders, most commonly Overanxious Disorder. Speech and language problems may contribute to the development of an Avoidant Disorder.

(Consult Checklist on page 26.)

AVOIDANT DISORDER OF
CHILDHOOD OR ADOLESCENCE
INTERVIEW FORM

1. Does the child show a desire for involvement with family members?

25

CHECKLIST

AVOIDANT DISORDER OF
CHILDHOOD OR ADOLESCENCE

Major Symptoms:

Key

-	Inattention
-	Impulsivity
-	Abnormal Activity Level
-	Aggressiveness
-	Violation of Rules
+	Isolation/Withdrawal/Avoidance
+	Inability to Form/Maintain Relationships
-	Disturbances of Affect or Mood
+	Anxiety
-	Depression
-	Delusions/Hallucinations
-	Somatic Complaints
-	Oddities of Behavior
*	Language Impairment
-	Impaired Cognition

Key
+ Presence
- Absence
* Associated Feature

Demographic Variables:

Age of Onset: After 2 and 1/2 years of age.
Duration: At least 6 months.

2. Does the child's avoidance of unfamiliar others interfere with the development of normal peer relationships?
3. How long has this pattern of social avoidance been evident and at what age did it begin?
4. Describe the child's behavior in situations with unfamiliar others.
5. Is the child easily embarrassed and/or timid when away from family members?
6. Are the child's communication skills significantly inhibited when in the presence of strangers?
7. Does the child have a history of speech and language impairment?

AVOIDANT DISORDER OF
CHILDHOOD OR ADOLESCENCE
CASE SUMMARY - Rick, C.A., 9-0

School Psychological Report/Reason for Referral: Rick was referred for an evaluation due to continuing concerns about his slow rate of academic progress and his insufficient participation in the academic setting. His functioning was characterized by intermittent periods of concentration on tasks and limited follow-through on assigned work. Additionally, Rick appeared to be easily overwhelmed by his social anxiety and fears of failure. His use of expressive language in the classroom setting was described as limited.

Background Information: Mother indicated that there was initial delay in Rick's acquisition of speech skills. There are no reported concerns with Rick's social interaction at home, where he is described as pleasant, cooperative, social, and independent. However, there is concern about Rick's lack of friends outside the home.

Mother reported that Rick began to demonstrate perfectionistic tendencies and social withdrawal while attending a nursery program when he was 3 years old. Recently she stated that Rick is verbalizing a number of fears, particularly when having to participate in social activities away from home.

Test Findings: Teacher's reports and observations in the classroom corroborated that, at times, Rick avoids answering or will only whisper when giving answers or when communicating with his teacher or peers.

Rick accompanied the examiner to the testing sessions without obvious reticence. He initiated no spontaneous verbalizations and responded to the examiner's attempts at conversation with minimal, often one-word responses. Rick occasionally displayed appropriate humor, though at a primitive level. In general, his affect was flat.

Rick presented himself as a highly anxious, threat-sensitive youngster. He responded to tasks only when directed, appearing not to risk providing more information than was specifically required. He took considerable time completing tasks. His initial responses to verbal items were often delayed.

Personality assessment suggested emotional constriction, dependency, and doubts regarding personal worth and belonging. Rick showed conflict and discomfort about what he knows is socially right and his inability to act appropriately on this knowledge. He continues to make excessive use of withdrawal and avoidance in coping with his anxieties. The extent of his use of these defense mechanisms constitutes a significant threat to healthy personality development.

Psychiatrist's Evaluation: Rick came to the interview willingly but quietly. He related with overt politeness but with very limited cooperativeness. He responded to questions with long silences and occasional, minimal verbal statements. His affect was constricted and was consistent with severe withdrawal.

I feel that Rick has an Avoidant Disorder. Although he is functioning with a mixture of strength and weakness, I feel that the pervasive use of avoidance and withdrawal is indicative of a serious emotional disorder. Major remediation lies in his receiving intensive outside psychotherapy.

The difficulties that Rick is experiencing academically derive from his internal, self-reinforcing psychodynamics. For this reason, I doubt that any changes could be made in the school setting that would significantly ameliorate the situation.

AUTHORS' COMMENTS

Rick presents himself as a highly anxious boy who deals with perceptions of threat from social situations by withdrawal and avoidance, to the extent of seriously affecting his communication, academic, and social skills.

Outside the home, he is inhibited and constricted, expressing doubts about his self-worth and fears of failure. He is also reported to have few friends. By contrast, at home Rick was described as independent and secure, and has warm relationships with family members.

Diagnosis of Avoidant Disorder was given because of Rick's excessive shrinking from social situations outside the home, particularly with peers, and the subsequent degree of impairment in his social functioning.

SOCIAL PHOBIA

There were no major changes made in the diagnostic criteria for Social Phobia from the *DSM-III* to the *DSM-III-R.*

The differences between Social Phobia and Avoidant Disorder of Childhood or Adolescence are subtle. In Avoidant Disorder, the essential feature is general shrinking from contact with unfamiliar people. In Social Phobia, avoidance may occur as a result of fear of scrutiny by others regarding behaviors or performance in a specific area. When outside of such situations, these individuals are able to function normally. In general, Avoidant Disorder tends to occur earlier in childhood while Social Phobia more often begins in later childhood or early adolescence, when there is increased emphasis on the social self.

In Social Phobia, individuals are fearful of being humiliated or embarrassed by something they may do in the presence of others. One of the most prevalent examples of Social Phobia involves speaking in public. Other examples of this disorder include the fear of tripping over something, saying something foolish, or being unable to respond to questions in social situations.

When these children anticipate or are exposed to a situation that they fear, intense anxiety ensues. Either the given situation is avoided altogether, or when it is confronted, symptoms such as sweating, panicky feelings, tachycardia, and breathing difficulties may occur. The level of anxiety usually increases because of awareness of these anxiety reactions, their excessive and unreasonable nature, and the feeling that others may notice such distress.

To meet diagnostic criteria for Social Phobia, the anxiety must be severe enough to impair social functioning, occupational activities, or relationships with others. A possible complication in this disorder is the abuse of alcohol and/or barbiturates, which may be used to cope with the anxiety-provoking situation.

(Consult Checklist on page 31.)

SOCIAL PHOBIA
INTERVIEW FORM

1. Has the person expressed fear about performance in social situations? Describe the specific situation where this occurs.
2. Has the person specifically avoided anxiety-provoking situations?
3. When confronted with the anxiety-provoking situation, how does the individual react?
4. Is the person aware that his or her fears are excessive and unreasonable given the situation?
5. To what degree does the avoidant behavior interfere with social or occupational functioning?
6. Does the person engage in the abuse of drugs to cope with the anxiety-provoking situation?
7. At what age did the avoidant behavior become evident?

SOCIAL PHOBIA
CASE SUMMARY - Jill, C.A., 15-0

Jill came to the school psychologist seeking help because of increasingly severe panic attacks when entering the school building. She stated that she has tried to reduce her anxiety by taking tranquilizers in the morning before school, and is considering not completing this semester.

Jill related that upon entering the school building she feels short of breath, begins to perspire, feels her heart racing, and has the urge to turn around and leave the grounds. Her daily schedule involves a speech and communication class during first period, where Jill is required to speak in public. She finds this increasingly threatening and anxiety provoking. She stated that she cannot speak as well as others and is afraid that class members will laugh at her attempts. Jill's fear has generalized to other classes when she is asked to participate verbally.

CHECKLIST

SOCIAL PHOBIA

Major Symptoms:

Key

-	Inattention
-	Impulsivity
-	Abnormal Activity Level
-	Aggressiveness
-	Violation of Rules
+	Isolation/Withdrawal/Avoidance
*	Inability to Form/Maintain Relationships
-	Disturbances of Affect or Mood
+	Anxiety
*	Depression
-	Delusions/Hallucinations
*	Somatic Complaints
-	Oddities of Behavior
-	Language Impairment
-	Impaired Cognition

Key
+ Presence
- Absence
* Associated Feature

Demographic Variables:

Age of Onset: Late childhood or early adolescence.
Duration: Usually chronic.

By contrast, Jill feels comfortable in talking informally with friends. She has tried practicing her speeches with them and at home with her family, where she does well. It is only when she has to perform for others that panic strikes.

Upon psychiatric consultation, a diagnosis of Social Phobia was made.

AUTHORS' COMMENTS

Jill's complaints meet the criteria for Social Phobia. When required to perform publicly she experiences panic and anxiety attacks. Her fears of embarrassment are specific to a given situation as she is able to function normally at most other times. Her attempts to remedy this situation by using drugs place her at risk for future drug abuse. Her self-referral to the school psychologist would suggest a good prognosis through therapy.

OVERANXIOUS DISORDER

Anxiety in this disorder resembles the Generalized Anxiety Disorder often found in adults, in that it is manifested by excessive or unrealistic worry about life events. In younger children, anxiety tends to be more focused, for example, preoccupation with a specific person perceived as overly critical or threatening. However, as they mature, anxiety becomes more diffused and permeates these children's judgments about peers, social relationships, academics, and athletic competence.

Anxiety generally involves an overall concern about performance and the opinion others may have of the individual's competency. It may center around future events, such as examinations, risk of injury, group acceptance, or meeting deadlines and expectations from others. At times, the appropriateness of past behaviors also elicits excessive concern. These children may have exaggerated worry about minor occurrences, such as routine visits to the doctor, and simple decision making regarding peers and family activities. They may become overly preoccupied with the judgment of others and complain that others are mean to them or are treating them unfairly.

Physical complaints associated with anxiety are often present and may take the form of nausea, headaches, dizziness, insomnia, or shortness of breath. Often there is motor restlessness, nail-biting, hair pulling, and other nervous habits. These children may complain of "feeling very nervous and unable to relax" and convey a general impression of tenseness.

Children with Overanxious Disorder are often described as overly mature, perfectionistic, and self-conscious. Because of their excessive self-doubts, they seek frequent reassurance and approval. In more severe cases, this disorder may include Social and Simple Phobia, in which these children become incapacitated to the extent of being unable to meet the demands of home and school. Although children with this disorder may refuse to attend school, this is not due to anxiety about separation from significant others (Separation Anxiety Disorder), but rather due to anxiety specifically concerning the school setting.

This disorder is reported to be more prevalent among oldest children of small families in the upper socio-economic levels, who may have high expectations and an overemphasis on achievement, even if actual performance is at an average or superior level.

(Consult Checklist on page 34.)

OVERANXIOUS DISORDER
INTERVIEW FORM

1. Does the child show persistent anxiety or worry about future events, such as examinations, possibility of injury, meeting expectations, or inclusion in a peer group?
2. Is he or she overly concerned about past behaviors?
3. Is he or she overly preoccupied about competence in academic, social, or athletic situations?
4. Does he or she show excessive need for reassurance?
5. Does he or she frequently complain of headaches, stomach pains, and other somatic concerns when there is no physical basis for such?
6. Does he or she seem easily embarrassed and self-conscious?
7. Does he or she seem unusually tense and unable to relax?
8. How long have any of these behaviors been observed?

CHECKLIST

OVERANXIOUS DISORDER

Major Symptoms:

Key

-	Inattention
-	Impulsivity
-	Abnormal Activity Level
-	Aggressiveness
-	Violation of Rules
*	Isolation/Withdrawal/Avoidance
*	Inability to Form/Maintain Relationships
-	Disturbances of Affect or Mood
+	Anxiety
-	Depression
-	Delusions/Hallucinations
+	Somatic Complaints
*	Oddities of Behavior
-	Language Impairment
-	Impaired Cognition

Key
+ Presence
- Absence
* Associated
  Feature

Demographic Variables:

Age of Onset: Before age 18.
Duration: At least 6 months.

34

9. Does the child exhibit any nervous habits such as nail-biting or restlessness, or has the child complained of feeling tense or nervous?
10. Does the child have difficulties falling asleep at night?
11. Does the child exhibit perfectionistic tendencies?
12. Does the child seek excessive reassurance because of persistent self-doubt?
13. Does the child express frequent complaints about peers and/or adults, and describe them as mean or overly critical?
14. What is the level of parental expectations for the child's achievement in social, academic, and other performance areas? How do these expectations compare to the child's actual functioning?

OVERANXIOUS DISORDER
CASE SUMMARY - Michael, C.A., 7-4

Reason for Referral: Michael's parents requested an evaluation to determine if their son has any special learning problems and to see if his tendency to withdraw should be given special attention. His school history reveals frequent absences over the past year.

Background History: Michael's parents are both college graduates. Michael is one of fraternal twins who, according to his parents, always has been developmentally behind his brother. His twin seems able to do everything quite well and Michael is in his "shadow" as a result. Both children are in 2nd grade and in the same classroom, as the school is small and there is no other 2nd grade.

There is no significant medical history, other than recurrent ear infections for which tubes were placed in Michael's eardrums 1 year earlier. Reports from school indicate frequent visits to the nurse's office because of complaints of headaches.

Evaluations: On examination, Michael was shy and withdrawn and eye contact was poor. He appeared nervous and tense throughout the evaluation, even when frequent feedback and reassurance were offered to him. Much erasing on paper and pencil tasks as well as overall dissatisfaction with his own production were noted.

A psychological evaluation revealed Superior intellectual functioning (FSIQ 123). The Bender was 1-1/2 years delayed. In educational testing, no major weaknesses were found other than in written performance.

Projective testing suggested a great deal of anxiety, tension, and self-criticism. Michael tended to internalize feelings and use fantasy and intellectualization rather than seek interaction with others. A strong tendency to use avoidance in stressful situations was noted, contributing to his high rate of absence from school. He was quite constricted in his emotional expression, using short phrases and speaking in a very soft tone.

Diagnosis: Overanxious Disorder.

Recommendations: Michael would benefit from systematic feedback and short-term assignments in a classroom setting where he would receive support and nonjudgmental reinforcement for his efforts. Tasks that would enhance his self-image and social standing in the classroom should be considered.

Further exploration of his academic achievement and expectations should be pursued with Michael's parents, preferably through family counseling. Less emphasis on academics and more time spent in noncompetitive, leisure activities at home would be of benefit.

AUTHORS' COMMENTS

Michael is experiencing anxiety and tension related to his performance and general competence. As a defense against anxiety, Michael self-criticizes, intellectualizes, and avoids stressful situations. Although of superior intelligence, he has become shy and withdrawn as a way of protecting himself from the judgment of others.

The fact that family counseling was recommended suggests that there may be pressures and expectations in the family that Michael feels unable to fulfill.

The clinical summary does not address Michael's social functioning. To rule out other disorders, it is important to determine his ability to seek and maintain peer relationships. Also unknown is the extent of his worry when dealing with other daily situations; therefore, we do not know if his anxiety is primarily school-oriented or pervades other occurrences in his life.

SEPARATION ANXIETY DISORDER

In this disorder, anxiety is specific to the separation from important others or from the familiar environment such as home. Its intensity may approximate panic, and such distress is beyond what is expected for the child's age.

When separated from important others, these children may experience intense fears about the well-being of parents or themselves; they often fantasize about possible accidents, serious illness, or traumatic events that may occur to themselves or those to whom they are attached. The identification of such fears usually gains in specificity as the child becomes older and more cognitively mature. When separation occurs, these children exhibit social withdrawal, apathy, and lack of involvement in play or work activities.

Children experiencing Separation Anxiety usually have sleep disturbances and frequent nightmares, and seek out their parents for reassurance. They may be fearful of animals, monsters, burglars, kidnappers, or the like. They may exhibit clinging behaviors inappropriate to their age, such as following a parent around the house. As a result of these fears, many children refuse to sleep at a friend's home or attend overnight camp.

When separation is anticipated or does occur, physical complaints are common, such as nausea, headaches, and vomiting. Besides psychosomatic involvement, violent aggressive behavior may occur towards those forcing separation.

Children with Separation Anxiety tend to behave in a demanding manner, seeking constant attention. Others may show unusual eagerness to please, conformity, and task-oriented behavior. Depression may accompany other symptoms of this disorder and become chronic over time. These children tend to come from close-knit, caring home environments. In many cases, the onset of this disorder follows a traumatic event in the child's life such as school change, the loss of a pet or family member, illness in the child or relative, or a move to new surroundings.

Although school refusal is usually part of a Separation Anxiety Syndrome, in this disorder anxiety occurs in a variety of situations in which the separation from important others is the key factor. By contrast, true school phobia involves specific fear of the school setting, regardless of the presence or absence of the parent.

CHECKLIST
SEPARATION ANXIETY DISORDER

Major Symptoms:

Key

-	Inattention		+ Presence
-	Impulsivity		- Absence
-	Abnormal Activity Level		* Associated
*	Aggressiveness		Feature
-	Violation of Rules		
+	Isolation/Withdrawal/Avoidance		
+	Inability to Form/Maintain Relationships		
-	Disturbances of Affect or Mood		
+	Anxiety		
*	Depression		
-	Delusions/Hallucinations		
+	Somatic Complaints		
-	Oddities of Behavior		
-	Language Impairment		
-	Impaired Cognition		

Demographic Variables:

Age of Onset: Before age 18.
Duration: At least 2 weeks.

SEPARATION ANXIETY DISORDER
INTERVIEW FORM

1. Does the child express unrealistic worry that something bad may happen to his or her family?
2. Does the child show clinging, shadowing behaviors towards important figure(s)?
3. Does he or she complain of nausea, headaches, or vomiting when away from or anticipating separation from important others?
4. Does he or she display temper tantrums, excessive crying, or panic reactions when parents are about to leave?
5. When away from the major attachment figure, does the child behave in a socially withdrawn, apathetic, sad manner?
6. Does he or she have nightmares with recurrent themes of being left alone?
7. Does the child refuse or is the child reluctant to sleep by him or herself or away from home?
8. Does he or she express unrealistic worry about animals or monsters; being lost, kidnapped, killed, or a victim of an accident?
9. Does he or she show a persistent pattern of school refusal in order to stay at home with parents?
10. How long have any of these behaviors been observed?
11. Has there been a recent traumatic event in the child's life, such as death, accident, serious illness, or a recent move to new surroundings?
12. Describe the child's behavior when separation from the major attachment figure is forced.
13. Does the child manifest signs of depression?

SEPARATION ANXIETY DISORDER
CASE SUMMARY - Lisa, C.A., 15-4

Reason for Referral: Lisa was referred for psychological evaluation to determine appropriate educational placement for the coming year.

Background Information: Lisa is presently placed in a homebound instruction program, originally recommended by a psychiatrist as a result of a series of traumatic experiences including physical and sexual assaults. There has been little progress in the program; her tutor indicates frequent interruptions and cancellations.

Observations: Lisa is an attractive 15-year-old girl, who is extremely anxious about having to return to her former school after an absence of over 8 months. Both Lisa and her mother were extremely apprehensive upon first meeting the evaluator, with mother indicating that she wished to be present during testing. Lisa alternated between periods of apparent calm and overt anxiety. She began to perspire inappropriately on several occasions and told the evaluator that she "just gets nervous for no reason."

Test Interpretation: Lisa's performance on the Rorschach and Thematic Apperception Test suggested a very insecure and anxious youngster overstriving to secure satisfaction from her environment. A high degree of anxiety content, such as fires, storm clouds, and explosions was present, as well as a persistent theme of violence indicative of her apparent phobic reaction to recent traumatic experiences. Lisa's drawing of a person depicted a small, nonintegrated, cartoon-like figure, and appeared to reflect a self-deprecatory attitude.

Psychiatric Evaluation: This mid-adolescent girl is experiencing a classic Separation Anxiety Disorder with school refusal. It arises from fears triggered by the physical and sexual assaults that occurred during the last school year. Her present Separation Anxiety and fears of leaving the security of home continue to play a part in Lisa's inability to cope with the reality of new encounters and involvement with other people.

While Lisa feels anxious about going to strange places where she feels assault is likely to recur, her anxiety centers around fears of separating from persons upon whom she is predominantly dependent. The separation anxiety is apparently nurtured by an overly protective maternal relationship. The anxiety is dissipated only as it is faced and encountered; consequently, one does not aid Lisa by allowing her to remain out of school. To the contrary, one only allows her, through manipulation, to perpetuate her state of internal anxiety and fear of separation.

Diagnosis: Separation Anxiety Disorder.

AUTHORS' COMMENTS

Lisa presents many of the features associated with Separation Anxiety: anxiety about going back to school, nervousness, insecurity, apprehension, fear about possible threatening events, and extreme dependency on others, specifically her mother. The fact that Lisa's mother asked to be present during the evaluation attests to their interdependency.

In Lisa's case, the onset of her separation anxiety seems to have been triggered by the series of recent assaults, which were highly traumatic for her.

POST-TRAUMATIC STRESS DISORDER

Post-Traumatic Stress Disorder differs from Adjustment Disorder in that in the latter, the stressor is usually not as severe and may be considered part of typical life experiences. In Post-Traumatic Stress Disorder, the stressor is significantly more serious and threatening, and is exceptional when compared to more typical stressors. Stressors of a mild nature which are more likely to result in a diagnosis of Adjustment Disorder may include such events as change of school, divorce, or birth of another sibling. More severe stressors resulting in the onset of Post-Traumatic Stress Disorder include devastating natural disasters, physical/sexual abuse, or witnessing the death of a parent. Although people experience all degrees of stressors, it is the individual's response to them that ultimately determines the presence of pathology, as well as the differential diagnosis between Adjustment Disorder and Post-Traumatic Stress Disorder.

This syndrome is manifested by symptoms associated with re-experiencing the traumatic event. Victims may recollect the traumatic event in such a vivid manner that they behave as if it were happening again, expressing the same anxiety and severe distress that accompanied the event the first time. In addition, they attempt to avoid thinking about the event, or avoid situations which may remind them of the trauma. For example, statements such as, "I don't want to talk about it," or "Don't remind me about it" are common.

Responses to such traumatic events usually begin with feelings of detachment, numbness, and subsequent withdrawal from people and activities once enjoyed. Specific behaviors may include disturbances of sleep patterns, angry outbursts, intensified states of alertness, impulsivity, depression, or loss of sustained concentration. In children, physical complaints such as headaches and stomachaches are common.

Young children may not be able to precisely identify the traumatic event but may, instead, demonstrate behaviors associated with it through play. In older children, statements indicating inability or lack of desire to project into the future may be common, such as, "I'll never marry," or "I'll never drive a car."

Onset of the symptoms of Post-Traumatic Stress Disorder may occur immediately, or from more than 6 months to several years after the traumatic event. Criteria for diagnosis are met when symptoms are present for at least 1 month. The diagnosis of this disorder also requires identification of the stressor, its degree of severity, and whether it is an acute event or an enduring situation.

(Consult Checklist on page 43.)

POST-TRAUMATIC STRESS DISORDER
INTERVIEW FORM

1. Has the child experienced a threatening or traumatic event? Please describe.
2. Does the child act as if he or she were re-experiencing the event by any of the following?

   a. Underlying distressing themes associated with the event through frequent verbal description or play.
   b. Distressing dreams associated with the event.
   c. Flashbacks, illusions, hallucinations, or actual behaviors that suggest that the child is re-experiencing the traumatic event.
   d. Significant distress with situations or circumstances that may symbolize or resemble the actual event.

CHECKLIST

POST-TRAUMATIC STRESS DISORDER

Major Symptoms:

Key

*	Inattention
*	Impulsivity
*	Abnormal Activity Level
*	Aggressiveness
-	Violation of Rules
+	Isolation/Withdrawal/Avoidance
*	Inability to Form/Maintain Relationships
*	Disturbances of Affect or Mood
+	Anxiety
*	Depression
*	Delusions/Hallucinations
*	Somatic Complaints
-	Oddities of Behavior
-	Language Impairment
-	Impaired Cognition

Key
+ Presence
- Absence
* Associated Feature

Demographic Variables:

Age of Onset: Any age, including childhood.
Duration: At least 1 month. Delayed onset is specified if the symptoms occur at least 6 months after the trauma.

3. Is the child avoiding specific stimuli, or is there a generalized bluntness of affect in his or her responses as characterized by any of the following?

    a. Denial or avoidance of thoughts and feelings associated with the event.
    b. Avoidance of situations that may remind him or her of the event.
    c. Inability to remember parts of the traumatic event.
    d. Decreased interest in previously enjoyed people and activities or regression to earlier developmental states, such as toilet training in young children.
    e. Feelings of disconnectedness from others.
    f. Diminished range of affective responses, such as the inability to give and/or receive affection.
    g. Expressed unwillingness to plan for the future.

4. Onset after the traumatic event of any of the following arousal symptoms:

    a. sleep disturbances
    b. irritability or angry outbursts
    c. decreased ability to concentrate
    d. intensified state of alertness
    e. easily alarmed
    f. Physiological responses when placed in a situation similar to or symbolizing an aspect of the event, such as perspiring or shortness of breath.

POST-TRAUMATIC STRESS DISORDER
CASE SUMMARY - Larry, C.A., 5-5

Reason for Referral: Larry's teacher was concerned about his high energy level, short attention span, inability to sit still and complete work independently, need for constant reassurance, and aggressive behavior towards others. In particular, Larry displays excessive attention-seeking behaviors. Academically, he appears to be capable of doing the work, but cannot accomplish anything if not given one-to-one attention.

Family and Social History: Larry is an only child. Mother reports a history of wife and child abuse by

Larry's father. He was the primary caretaker during infancy while the mother worked two jobs. The physical abuse incurred by Larry was primarily aimed at his legs, lower body, and backside. He was also reportedly tied to a chair with his mouth taped and put in a closet alone for hours at a time.

Mother notes that Larry exhibits a quick temper, stubbornness, and aggressiveness towards others. At other times, Larry appears sullen for no particular reason. He also has many fears. At home he follows his mother around and needs constant reassurance.

Clinical Assessment: Larry's intellectual functioning is at least in the High Average range. There is a large discrepancy between cognitive and emotional functioning.

During the evaluation, Larry made little eye contact, kept his voice quite loud, and often attempted to leave his seat. Projective testing had an extremely immature quality to it with signs of emotional lability, aggressive attitudes, and a high level of anxiety. There were themes of hostility, sadness, and fears of harm and rejection.

Psychiatric Consultation: Larry came to the interview willingly. He sat fairly still in his chair while he talked almost incessantly. He related in a very engaging, lively manner, and was most open and cooperative.

Larry's vocabulary was precocious, as was his capacity for comprehension and concept formation. At the same time, the content of his speech was rambling and rather confused. He claimed that he occasionally hears voices but it was difficult to determine the significance of that statement. He admitted that he occasionally feels sad but denied any suicidal feelings. He was able to describe some of the physical abuse that he experienced in the past at the hands of his father.

Larry is experiencing a Post-Traumatic Stress Disorder, secondary to his having been physically abused in the past. He is also very disorganized and erratic. The combination of these problems constitutes serious emotional disturbance. Consideration should be made for a special classroom placement for children with emotional disorders. Larry's chance to recover from his present emotional difficulties strongly depends upon family therapy.

AUTHORS' COMMENTS

Larry's history of abuse constitutes a severe traumatic event. Although this occurred several years ago, he still manifests many of the symptoms associated with this trauma; specifically anxiety, angry outbursts, depression, impulsivity, and loss of sustained concentration. Hallucinations may be present. Larry's symbolic recollection of being forced to remain in a chair with his mouth taped may manifest itself by his inability to sit still and his incessant talking while seated.

Other areas that could have been productively explored include Larry's sleep patterns, and social interactions outside of school. The report noted that Larry experiences significant fears but did not address their content. However, considering the major stressor and Larry's subsequent behaviors, the diagnosis of Post-Traumatic Stress Disorder appears appropriate.

ADDITIONAL READINGS
FOR ANXIETY DISORDERS

Beck, A. T., Emery, G. with Greenberg, R. (1985). *Anxiety Disorders and Phobias: A Cognitive Perspective.* New York: Basic Books.

Bowlby, J. (1980). *Attachment and Loss.* New York: Basic Books.

Edward, J., Ruskin, N., & Turrini, P. (1981). *Separation-Individuation: Theory and Application.* New York: Gardner Press.

Eth, S., & Pynoos, R. S. (Eds.). (1985). *Post-Traumatic Stress Disorder in Children.* Washington, DC: American Psychiatric Press.

Gaudry, E. (1971). *Anxiety and Educational Achievement.* New York: John Wiley.

Gewirtz, J. L. (Ed.). (1972). *Attachment and Dependency.* Washington: Winston.

Gittelman, R. (Ed.). (1986). *Anxiety Disorders of Childhood.* New York: John Wiley.

King, N. J. (1988). *Children's Phobias: A Behavioral Perspective.* New York: John Wiley.

Morris, R. J., & Kratochwill, T. R. (1983). *Treating Children's Fears and Phobias: A Behavioral Approach.* New York: Pergamon.

ADJUSTMENT DISORDERS

INTRODUCTION

Adjustment Disorder involves impairment of overall functioning, such as school or social activity, due to an excessive, maladaptive reaction occurring within 3 months of the onset of a stressful event.

In normal reactions to stressful situations, individuals tend to over-react and then recover. With an Adjustment Disorder, they continue to be significantly affected and do not return to their previous level of functioning without intervention. This intervention may involve either the removal of the given stressor(s) or assistance in developing coping mechanisms.

Stressors may be single or multiple, recurrent or continuous. Some stressors are associated with developmental stages such as the onset of adolescence; others with situational difficulties such as changing schools, neighborhoods, and so on. Stressors may involve familial events such as parental conflict, divorce, illness, or arrival of a newborn sibling. Other events that may affect individuals or entire communities include natural disasters or societal strife, such as racial or religious prejudice.

The severity of the stressor is specific to the individual situation and depends on the duration and time of life at which it occurs. Vulnerability to any stressor depends on the psychological make-up of the individual. Some are severely affected by a mild stressor, while others only experience mild adjustment disorders in the presence of significant stressors.

To arrive at a diagnosis of Adjustment Disorder, school personnel or other professionals need to be particularly careful in identifying the premorbid functioning of the child and the particular stressful event(s) triggering the change in behavior. Without this information, there may be an erroneous diagnosis such as Affective Disorder, Conduct Disorder, or Anxiety Disorder, due to the absence of crucial differential data.

The *DSM-III-R* identifies several types of Adjustment Disorders depending on the predominant symptoms at the time of referral.

ADJUSTMENT DISORDER WITH DEPRESSED MOOD

Predominant symptoms include depressed mood, hopelessness, and tearfulness.

ADJUSTMENT DISORDER WITH ANXIOUS MOOD

Predominant symptoms include worry, nervousness, and jitteriness.

ADJUSTMENT DISORDER WITH DISTURBANCE OF CONDUCT

Predominant symptoms include violations of the rights of others or of age-appropriate societal norms and rules.

ADJUSTMENT DISORDER WITH WITHDRAWAL

Predominant symptoms include withdrawal from social situations when previous social functioning was adequate.

ADJUSTMENT DISORDER WITH PHYSICAL COMPLAINTS

Predominant symptoms include physiological complaints such as fatigue, headaches, and other aches and pains.

ADJUSTMENT DISORDER WITH WORK OR ACADEMIC INHIBITION

Predominant symptoms involve the inability to work or function academically when previous performance was appropriate. Individuals may be unable to study or produce homework, papers, or reports. Usually a combination of anxiety and depression are also present.

ADJUSTMENT DISORDER WITH
MIXED EMOTIONAL FEATURES

Predominant symptoms include various combinations of depression and anxiety or other emotions.

ADJUSTMENT DISORDER WITH MIXED
DISTURBANCE OF EMOTIONS AND CONDUCT

Predominant features include various combinations of depression and anxiety as well as disturbance of conduct.

(Consult Checklists on pages 56-63.)

ADJUSTMENT DISORDERS
INTERVIEW FORM

1. Within the past 3 months, has the child been exposed to a significant stressful event(s) in his or her life? Describe.
2. Is there significant impairment in school, social, or occupational functioning?
3. Are the child's reactions excessive and/or uncommon given the particular stressor?
4. Has the child shown a similar behavioral pattern prior to the event(s)?
5. Does the child have a long-term tendency to overreact to stressful situations?
6. For how long have these symptoms been evident?
7. Has the child previously been diagnosed as having another mental disorder?

ADJUSTMENT DISORDER
CASE SUMMARY - Carl, C.A., 13-1

Reason for Referral: Carl was referred because of an abrupt change in his behavior 4 months ago. He was always a restless, somewhat rebellious child in the classroom, but recently his behavior has deteriorated significantly. He now becomes agitated at minimal provocation, has been throwing things, and tried to strangle one of his peers.

Interview with Parents: Both parents attended for this interview. We talked about mother's injuries; she was injured at work, treated at an intensive care unit, and seen by many neurologists. She had a subdural hematoma which was surgically treated. Following this, she developed a seizure, was placed on medication at the hospital, and then was released. Sometime later she discontinued medication and subsequently had another seizure. Mother admitted that she had become depressed due to a massive weight gain since the accident. She saw a psychiatrist, was hospitalized, and is currently taking anticonvulsive medication. Mother admitted that she was still depressed over her failure to lose weight. Neither parent seemed able to talk to Carl very effectively. Both of them were at a loss to understand his behavioral deterioration.

Interview with Carl: At first Carl denied any knowledge of stress at home, but he gradually became more verbal. He had witnessed his mother's original seizure and had been terrified. Carl described in detail how she began to shake, reached out for him, bit her tongue which bled, and had difficulties breathing. The boy was convinced that his mother was going to die. When she was initially hospitalized after her accident, Carl was aware that they had to "cut her head open and work on her brain." He was also aware of her second hospitalization with "bad nerves," and linked both incidents, becoming convinced that she was in mortal danger of dying.

Carl also spoke freely about conditions at home; his parents are always yelling at each other. According to him this is nothing new, as they have been fighting with each other for years. He is scared that one of them is going to leave, and spends his time worrying about this and about his mother's health.

Summary: Carl is obviously reacting to a number of stresses. He has developed persistent fear of his mother's dying based on inaccurate knowledge about seizures. Additionally, he is fearful of being abandoned by one or the other of his parents. Carl is a boy continually beset by worries, some of which can be resolved in counseling.

Diagnosis: Adjustment Disorder with Mixed Emotional Features.

Recommendations: Carl would benefit from a special education class for children with emotional problems, together with counseling intervention. Both parents should be seen to help them work things out with Carl in a frank and open manner, and to leave Carl with the impression that he will not be abandoned by one or both of his parents. Reassurance about his mother's physical condition can only occur after Carl is provided with a thorough explanation of the nature and outcome of her seizure disorder.

AUTHORS' COMMENTS

Before the onset of this disorder, Carl was described as a rebellious child, but not to the extent and severity demonstrated by his current behavior. Although several stressors were identified, the one that probably precipitated his change in behavior was witnessing his mother's seizure, which he could not fully understand. Fear of abandonment (through death or separation) became a preoccupation for him to the point of impairing his social and academic functioning. Emotional features operating at this time include a high degree of anxiety, anger, and depression. Based on this information, Carl is experiencing an Adjustment Disorder with Mixed Emotional Features.

ADDITIONAL READINGS
FOR ADJUSTMENT DISORDERS

Chandler, L. A. (1985). *Children Under Stress: Understanding Emotional Adjustment Reactions* (2nd ed.). Springfield, IL: Thomas.

Field, T., McCabe, P., & Schneiderman, N. (Eds.). (1985). *Stress and Coping.* Hillsdale, NJ: L. Erlbaum Associates.

Garmezy, N., & Rutter, M. (Eds.). (1983). *Stress, Coping, and Development in Children.* New York: McGraw-Hill.

CHECKLIST

ADJUSTMENT DISORDER
WITH DEPRESSED MOOD

Major Symptoms:

Key

*	Inattention
-	Impulsivity
-	Abnormal Activity Level
-	Aggressiveness
-	Violation of Rules
-	Isolation/Withdrawal/Avoidance
*	Inability to Form/Maintain Relationships
+	Disturbances of Affect or Mood
-	Anxiety
+	Depression
-	Delusions/Hallucinations
-	Somatic Complaints
-	Oddities of Behavior
-	Language Impairment
-	Impaired Cognition

Key

+ Presence

- Absence

* Associated Feature

Demographic Variables:

Age of Onset: Any age.
Duration: Begins within 3 months of onset of stressor, and lasts no longer than 6 months. Generally depends on the degree of severity of the stressor.

CHECKLIST

ADJUSTMENT DISORDER
WITH ANXIOUS MOOD

Major Symptoms:

Key

*	Inattention
-	Impulsivity
-	Abnormal Activity Level
-	Aggressiveness
-	Violation of Rules
-	Isolation/Withdrawal/Avoidance
*	Inability to Form/Maintain Relationships
+	Disturbances of Affect or Mood
+	Anxiety
-	Depression
-	Delusions/Hallucinations
-	Somatic Complaints
-	Oddities of Behavior
-	Language Impairment
-	Impaired Cognition

Key

+ Presence

- Absence

* Associated
  Feature

Demographic Variables:

Age of Onset: Any age.
Duration: Begins within 3 months of onset of stressor, and lasts no longer than 6 months. Generally depends on the degree of severity of the stressor.

57

CHECKLIST

ADJUSTMENT DISORDER
WITH DISTURBANCE OF CONDUCT

Major Symptoms:

*	Inattention
*	Impulsivity
-	Abnormal Activity Level
*	Aggressiveness
+	Violation of Rules
-	Isolation/Withdrawal/Avoidance
*	Inability to Form/Maintain Relationships
-	Disturbances of Affect or Mood
-	Anxiety
-	Depression
-	Delusions/Hallucinations
-	Somatic Complaints
-	Oddities of Behavior
-	Language Impairment
-	Impaired Cognition

Key

+ Presence
- Absence
* Associated Feature

Demographic Variables:

Age of Onset: Any age.
Duration: Begins within 3 months of onset of stressor, and lasts no longer than 6 months. Generally depends on the degree of severity of the stressor.

58

CHECKLIST

ADJUSTMENT DISORDER
WITH WITHDRAWAL

Major Symptoms:

Key

*	Inattention
-	Impulsivity
-	Abnormal Activity Level
-	Aggressiveness
-	Violation of Rules
+	Isolation/Withdrawal/Avoidance
*	Inability to Form/Maintain Relationships
-	Disturbances of Affect or Mood
-	Anxiety
-	Depression
-	Delusions/Hallucinations
-	Somatic Complaints
-	Oddities of Behavior
-	Language Impairment
-	Impaired Cognition

Key

+ Presence

- Absence

* Associated
  Feature

Demographic Variables:

Age of Onset: Any age.
Duration: Begins within 3 months of onset of stressor, and lasts no longer than 6 months. Generally depends on the degree of severity of the stressor.

59

CHECKLIST

ADJUSTMENT DISORDER
WITH PHYSICAL COMPLAINTS

Major Symptoms:

Key

*	Inattention
-	Impulsivity
-	Abnormal Activity Level
-	Aggressiveness
-	Violation of Rules
-	Isolation/Withdrawal/Avoidance
*	Inability to Form/Maintain Relationships
-	Disturbances of Affect or Mood
*	Anxiety
-	Depression
-	Delusions/Hallucinations
+	Somatic Complaints
-	Oddities of Behavior
-	Language Impairment
-	Impaired Cognition

Key:
+ Presence
- Absence
* Associated Feature

Demographic Variables:

Age of Onset: Any age.
Duration: Begins within 3 months of onset of stressor, and lasts no longer than 6 months. Generally depends on the degree of severity of the stressor.

CHECKLIST

ADJUSTMENT DISORDER WITH
WORK OR ACADEMIC INHIBITION

Major Symptoms:

Key

*	Inattention
-	Impulsivity
-	Abnormal Activity Level
-	Aggressiveness
-	Violation of Rules
-	Isolation/Withdrawal/Avoidance
-	Inability to Form/Maintain Relationships
*	Disturbances of Affect or Mood
*	Anxiety
*	Depression
-	Delusions/Hallucinations
-	Somatic Complaints
-	Oddities of Behavior
-	Language Impairment
-	Impaired Cognition

Key
+ Presence
- Absence
* Associated Feature

Demographic Variables:

Age of Onset: Any age.
Duration: Begins within 3 months of onset of stressor, and lasts no longer than 6 months. Generally depends on the degree of severity of the stressor.

61

CHECKLIST

ADJUSTMENT DISORDER WITH MIXED EMOTIONAL FEATURES

Major Symptoms:

Key

*	Inattention
-	Impulsivity
-	Abnormal Activity Level
-	Aggressiveness
-	Violation of Rules
-	Isolation/Withdrawal/Avoidance
*	Inability to Form/Maintain Relationships
+	Disturbances of Affect or Mood
*	Anxiety
*	Depression
-	Delusions/Hallucinations
-	Somatic Complaints
-	Oddities of Behavior
-	Language Impairment
-	Impaired Cognition

Key
+ Presence
- Absence
* Associated Feature

Demographic Variables:

Age of Onset: Any age.
Duration: Begins within 3 months of onset of stressor, and lasts no longer than 6 months. Generally depends on the degree of severity of the stressor.

CHECKLIST

ADJUSTMENT DISORDER WITH MIXED DISTURBANCE OF EMOTIONS AND CONDUCT

Major Symptoms:

Key

*	Inattention
*	Impulsivity
-	Abnormal Activity Level
*	Aggressiveness
+	Violation of Rules
-	Isolation/Withdrawal/Avoidance
*	Inability to Form/Maintain Relationships
+	Disturbances of Affect or Mood
*	Anxiety
*	Depression
-	Delusions/Hallucinations
-	Somatic Complaints
-	Oddities of Behavior
-	Language Impairment
-	Impaired Cognition

Key
+ Presence
- Absence
* Associated Feature

Demographic Variables:

Age of Onset: Any age.
Duration: Begins within 3 months of onset of stressor, and lasts no longer than 6 months. Generally depends on the degree of severity of the stressor.

PERVASIVE DEVELOPMENTAL DISORDERS

INTRODUCTION

In the *DSM-III*, this category of disorders included the syndromes of Infantile Autism and Childhood Onset Pervasive Developmental Disorder. The major differential diagnosis pertained to the age of onset: Infantile Autism, before 30 months; Childhood Onset Pervasive Developmental Disorder, after 30 months of age.

The *DSM-III* considered the distinction between Infantile Autism, Childhood Onset Pervasive Developmental Disorder, and Schizophrenia in children a controversial issue but opted for the separation of these three disorders. The difference focused primarily on the presence or absence of delusions, hallucinations, and loosening of associations. However, the determination of such symptoms in young children was reportedly difficult to assess.

The *DSM-III-R* no longer differentiates among subcategories of the general classification of Pervasive Developmental Disorders because they all share a common core of disturbance. The major diagnosis is Autistic Disorder. There is also a category of Pervasive Developmental Disorder Not Otherwise Specified to be considered when the criteria for Autistic Disorder are not met because of qualitative differences.

Partly because of the difficulty in documenting the presence of delusions and hallucinations in children, the *DSM-III-R* does not include the term psychosis as part of Autistic Disorder. Therefore, Childhood Schizophrenia is not included as a subcategory of Pervasive Developmental Disorders. It may, however, share many of the symptoms associated with Autistic Disorder, such as withdrawal, peculiar behavior, and inappropriate affect.

Age of Onset, which was an important distinction between Infantile Autism and Childhood Onset Pervasive Developmental Disorder in the *DSM-III*, is no longer a criteria for differentiation in the *DSM-III-R*. It recognizes the difficulties in obtaining reliable estimates of onset because of parental inexperience and/or uncertainty.

However, in the great majority of cases, onset can be identified by age 3.

AUTISTIC DISORDER

Both Autistic Disorder and Pervasive Developmental Disorder Not Otherwise Specified share common symptoms but vary in the degree in which they are manifested; Autistic Disorder being the more severe of the two. Behavioral characteristics of this disorder include the following:

QUALITATIVE IMPAIRMENT IN RECIPROCAL SOCIAL INTERACTION

Interaction with others shows failure to form attachments, and overall lack of interest in people since infancy. This is usually demonstrated by minimum eye contact, unresponsiveness, or aversion to cuddling, affection, and physical contact. In early childhood, there is failure to develop cooperative, imaginative play, or social friendships. Depending on the degree of impairment and age of these children, they may eventually appear to demonstrate some social interest. However, this is considered a shallow attempt and does not reflect true social interaction.

QUALITATIVE IMPAIRMENT IN VERBAL AND NONVERBAL COMMUNICATION, AND IMAGINATIVE ACTIVITY

Deficits in communication involve verbal and nonverbal abilities. If language is present, children with this disorder show echolalia, unusual speech melodies, lack of abstract terms, poor syntactic structure, word meanings usually known only to themselves, and difficulties in naming familiar objects. The usual expected facial expressions and gestures are either absent or inappropriate. When older, there is inability to comprehend jokes, irony, and double meanings.

In the area of imaginative activity, children with this disorder lack the type of flexible, make-believe play requiring fantasy and imagination. When playing, they are observed engaging in the same repetitive activities without change or variety.

MARKEDLY RESTRICTED REPERTOIRE
OF ACTIVITIES AND INTERESTS

Abnormal responses to the environment can take many forms; the child may resist minor changes, and be obsessively interested in specific objects, music, movement, or parts of the body. For example, the child may react violently to a simple change in routine, such as change of placement of a toy, or sequence in dressing or washing. Adults may notice an excessive attachment to such unusual objects as buttons and rubber bands, or obsessive attraction to a specific sound.

OTHER FEATURES

These children have frequent and unexplainable mood changes ranging from laughing to crying. There is lack of sensitivity or oversensitivity to such sensory stimuli as light, sound, or pain. They often seem unaware of such possible dangers as heights or street traffic or become overly fearful and tense when encountering innocuous objects or events. Repetitive and peculiar motor movements such as handclapping, twirling, and spinning, are often observed in children with this disorder. Additional abnormalities may include self-mutilation or other self-damaging behaviors such as biting, head banging, and the like. Parents may report unusual patterns of eating, sleeping, and drinking; for example, a limited diet by the child's own choice, or excessive fluid intake.

Significant delays in cognitive skills are evident in this syndrome. If testable, these children usually show better performance on manipulative tasks as opposed to abstract, verbal abilities. Some children may have an unusual long-term memory of isolated information, retained over several years. Despite the presence of scatter skills, these children commonly test in the Moderate to Severe range of mental retardation.

Predisposing physiological factors associated with Pervasive Developmental Disorders are maternal rubella, phenylketonuria, anoxia during birth, encephalitis, and infantile seizures. In controlled studies, parental personality and/or characteristics in the interaction with the child have not been found to be predisposing factors for these disorders.

CHECKLIST

AUTISTIC DISORDER

Major Symptoms:

		Key
*	Inattention	+ Presence
*	Impulsivity	- Absence
*	Abnormal Activity Level	* Associated Feature
-	Aggressiveness	
-	Violation of Rules	
-	Isolation/Withdrawal/Avoidance	
+	Inability to Form/Maintain Relationships	
+	Disturbances of Affect or Mood	
-	Anxiety	
-	Depression	
-	Delusions/Hallucinations	
-	Somatic Complaints	
+	Oddities of Behavior	
+	Language Impairment	
+	Impaired Cognition	

Demographic Variables:

Age of Onset: Infancy or childhood.
Duration: Chronic.

70

AUTISTIC DISORDER
INTERVIEW FORM

The following questions have been separated into the three major symptom categories described previously: Qualitative Impairment in Reciprocal Social Interaction; Qualitative Impairment in Verbal and Nonverbal Communication, and Imaginative Activity; and Markedly Restricted Repertoire of Activities and Interests. Within each symptom category, the questions have been arranged from younger or more severe to older or less severe manifestations of this disorder (*DSM-III-R*).

Qualitative Impairment in Reciprocal Social Interaction:

1. Does the child show significant lack of awareness of the existence or feelings of others?
2. Does the child seek comfort when ill, hurt, or tired? Describe.
3. Does the child imitate normal routines of others? Describe.
4. Does the child participate in social play activities?
5. Does the child show understanding of the rules and conventions of social interaction?

Qualitative Impairment in Verbal and NonVerbal Communication, and Imaginative Play:

6. Does the child use age-appropriate communication skills such as babbling, facial expression, mimicking, or spoken language?
7. Does the child use age-appropriate nonverbal communication, such as eye-gaze, facial expression, body posture, and in general, gestures to initiate or respond to interaction?
8. Does the child engage in imaginative activities such as using fantasy, play acting, or imaginary characters?
9. Does the child have peculiarities of speech such as lack of variety in tone of voice, inappropriate pitch and volume, or statements ending in question-like melodies?
10. Does the child show significant impairment in speech form and content, such as echolalia, repet-

itive use of speech, inappropriate use of pronouns, or irrelevancy of subject matter?

11. Does the child show significant impairment in his or her ability to initiate conversation and maintain dialogue?

Markedly Restricted Repertoire of Activities and Interests:

12. Does the child show odd motor movements such as unusual hand-finger movements, spinning, walking on tiptoes, or head-banging?
13. Is the child overly preoccupied with smells, parts of objects, textures of things, spinning wheels of toy cars; or is he or she overly attached to uncommon objects, such as string or rubber bands?
14. Is he or she unable to cope with minor everyday changes in the environment?
15. Does he or she have a compulsive need to do things in the same manner everyday?
16. Does the child show a restricted range of interests; for instance, interest only in lining up objects, collecting facts about one subject, or pretending to be an imaginary character?
17. At what age were these behaviors first observed?
18. Is the child over or undersensitive to such stimuli as sound or light?
19. Does the child experience extreme mood swings such as unexplained crying, giggling, or laughing?
20. Does the child respond appropriately to real dangers in the environment such as traffic or heights?
21. Has a recent audiogram ruled out deafness?
22. Have there been attempts at psychological testing? If so, what are the results?
23. Does the family history indicate any serious maternal health problems during pregnancy such as rubella?
24. Has the child ever had any serious illnesses, for instance, encephalitis?

AUTISTIC DISORDER
CASE SUMMARY - Gary, C.A., 6-0

Referral Reason: Gary's parents initiated the referral and requested an unbiased opinion of Gary's problems. Information from other sources, except neurological and audiological examinations, was not available to the present examiners.

Background Information: Gary, the oldest of two children, was born weighing 6 pounds, 9 ounces, by Cesarean section, without any maternal problems except for some mild toxemic symptoms. His mother describes her pregnancy with Gary as a very difficult one. She was under the care of a physician for the entire time, with frequent nausea, dizziness, blackouts, and high blood pressure. She was hospitalized at 5 months, at which time she felt physicians were indicating that she might wish to consider a voluntary abortion. She refused to think of that possibility and continued through the pregnancy.

From birth to the age of 3 months, there were some serious feeding problems. Gary vomited frequently. He was not gaining weight and was unable to keep his feedings down. Gary never slept much as an infant; as a result, his parents also found it difficult to sleep. He was never on a schedule, which was very aggravating to his mother.

When he was 2 years of age, things settled down somewhat, and Gary went on to more of a routine. Developmental milestones in some areas are unremarkable. Gary was sitting with help between 4 and 5 months, and alone at 6 months. He never crawled, but went from sitting to walking with help at 10 months, and alone at 12 months. He was toilet trained for daytime at about 3-1/2 years; at nighttime he is still not bladder trained. His mother had a good deal of difficulty in training Gary and managed only because she "kept after him constantly."

Gary was babbling at 6 months of age. He stopped making sounds a few weeks before his first birthday, when he began to walk. He made no more sounds until he was about 3 to 3-1/2 years old. There were never any single recognizable words, combined words, or sentences. Gary is not interested in looking at books except to rip them. He has no interest in being read to, either.

Developmentally, his mother feels that some days, with the exception of speech, Gary seems to do things "normally." Other days, and these are most of the time, he has some problems following directions, amusing himself, and functioning in matters of daily living.

Health History: As a small baby Gary was always sick with colds, fever, earaches, or "something." He had a high fever, and from the description it sounds as though there was a convulsion. Until the age of 2 or 2-1/2, he had frequent ear infections and running ears. A recent audiological examination ruled out any hearing impairment.

Parents report that Gary's favorite activities are playing on his swings, finger painting, and cutting with scissors. He makes his needs known mostly by helping himself to whatever he desires. For example, if he wants a drink and someone else has a drink of something on the table, he will take that other person's glass and drink from it. When he can't explain himself or make his needs known, he gets terribly frustrated and will kick and throw.

When he was here, we noted some activity with his fingers, which his parents later explained as starting when attempts were made to begin teaching him sign language. Prior to that time, Gary showed no unusual finger concentration.

Psychological Assessment: Gary's interactions with people and objects have been extremely limited. He has numerous toys but seldom plays with them. He enjoys swings and will, on occasion, watch one or two cartoons on television. Gary appears to have limited awareness of his 17-month-old sibling, and will often push him out of his way or just walk into him.

According to his parents, when Gary was approximately 3 years of age he said, "I want a drink." This was the first and last sentence they heard. He will occasionally say "mommy" when in distress but generally emits numerous unspecific sounds.

Gary has frequent temper tantrums whenever he is frustrated in obtaining something he wants, engages in lengthy staring spells while rocking, and spends considerable time tearing the pages of books. Also reported and evidenced throughout the evaluation was ritualistic, compulsive fingerplay.

Gary withdrew when he initially met the examiner. His contact, such as holding hands while walking to the test room, was marked by indifference or almost total lack of awareness of people or surroundings. Impulsivity predominated throughout the evaluation session. Gary was unable to focus on any material and use it adaptively. He moved from object to object without meaningfully using it.

Gary's limited exploration of materials was on a very primitive level. He would smell materials presented to him, then put them down and begin engaging in finger posturing. When further attempts were made to have him investigate materials, he would generally mouth them. Hand puppets were presented but they did not elicit appropriate behavior. Although there was an increase in the sounds he made, he generally pushed them away or bit their heads.

Attempts to have Gary carry out commands proved futile for the most part. However, on two occasions he was able to follow through when demands were repeated at a rapid pace. At these times however, there was noticeable increase in his activity level, finger posturing, and the appearance of spinning behavior. Gary twirled himself around as he approached the object he was asked to obtain.

Impressions: Gary demonstrated gross and sustained impairment of emotional relationships with people. He is unaware of his own personal identity to a degree appropriate for his age. He appears to have little to no regard for the accepted function of objects in his environment, and demonstrates a sustained resistance to change in his environment. Speech appears to have been acquired but then lost, and his parents cite numerous developmental problems. All of these behaviors are indicative of Autism. I suggest that approaches to Gary and his development be modeled after those used with autistic children.

AUTHORS' COMMENTS

With respect to Qualitative Impairment in Reciprocal Social Interaction, Gary shows significant lack of awareness of people and his surroundings with almost no responsivity towards them.

Language development, if in fact it occurred at all, is currently reduced to unspecific sounds and does not appear related to any attempts at communication. Additionally, there is little evidence of Imaginative Play, as demonstrated by his inability to creatively use puppets, for example.

Gary evidenced rocking, spinning, twirling, finger concentration, and other ritualistic behaviors symptomatic of Restricted Activities and Interests. His inability to respond appropriately involved such behaviors as book ripping, grabbing items from others, and not responding to any requests.

An audiological examination ruled out hearing loss which might have contributed to delayed language acquisition. A formal psychological evaluation could not be completed due to Gary's lack of responsivity; he smelled and mouthed the test materials.

Given these behaviors and the degree and severity of Gary's impairment, the diagnosis of Autistic Disorder has been appropriately made.

ADDITIONAL READINGS FOR
PERVASIVE DEVELOPMENTAL DISORDERS

Cohen, D., & Donnellan, A. M. (Eds.). (1987). *Handbook of Autism and Pervasive Developmental Disorders.* New York: John Wiley.

Groden, G., & Baron, M. G. (Eds.). (1988). *Autism: Strategies for Change: A Comprehensive Approach to the Education and Treatment of Children with Autism and Related Disorders.* New York: Gardner Press.

Schreibman, L. E. (1988). *Autism.* Newbury Park, CA: Sage.

Steffen, J. J., & Karoly, P. (Eds.). (1982). *Autism and Severe Child Psychopathology.* Lexington, MA: Lexington Books.

OTHER DISORDERS OF CHILDHOOD AND ADOLESCENCE

SCHIZOPHRENIA

The general description of symptoms associated with Schizophrenia has remained for the most part unchanged in the revision of the *DSM-III*. The diagnostic criteria, however, have been reorganized to address the symptoms required for inclusion in the diagnosis of Schizophrenia.

The *DSM-III-R* considers Schizophrenia a group of disorders, all of which present symptoms involving multiple psychological processes, deterioration from highest level of previous functioning, duration of at least 6 months, and onset usually before mid-life.

SYMPTOMS INVOLVING MULTIPLE PSYCHOLOGICAL PROCESSES

The following disturbances in psychological processes are also found in other disorders; no single characteristic pertains exclusively to Schizophrenia, but at least one must be present for the diagnosis of Schizophrenia.

Content of Thought: The primary disturbance in the content of these individuals' thinking involves delusions not based on reality. Delusions can be either multiple, bizarre, or fragmented. Among the most common are: thought broadcasting (the belief that other people can hear their thoughts), thought insertion (the belief that others are placing thoughts into their mind), thought withdrawal (the belief that someone has removed thoughts from their mind), and delusions of being controlled (the belief that they don't own their own thoughts, but that these are being controlled by outside forces). Other delusions include feelings of persecution, delusions of reference (in which these individuals place unusual significance on common objects, people, or events in the belief that such are harmful or insulting to them). Thinking marked by contradictions, erroneous conclusions (given the initial statement), and overvaluation of habits, particular activities, and the like may also be present.

Form of Thought: In addition to disturbances in the content of thought, Schizophrenia is also characterized by disturbed thinking and the unawareness of its lack of cohesiveness. Unconnected ideas, loosening of associations, and shifting from one topic to the next are common. At such times speech may become unintelligible, stereotyped, excessively abstract or concrete; although these individuals appear to generate vast verbal output, a closer look at its content reveals a lack of logic, cohesiveness, and information.

Perception: All forms of hallucinations can be found in this disorder, particularly those of an auditory nature. Single or multiple voices, usually of a critical nature, are perceived as coming into the head from the outside. Some of these auditory hallucinations may be commanding and dangerous if these individuals act upon them.

Hallucinations may involve all senses: tactile, visual, gustatory, olfactory, and kinesthetic. However, if these occur without the presence of auditory hallucinations, an organic mental disorder should be considered.

Affect: Disturbances of affect are difficult to detect unless they appear in an extreme form. Types of disturbed affect may include blunting (reduced intensity of affective expression), flat affect (absence of affective expression, i.e., expressionless face, monotonous voice), and inappropriate affect (affect in blatant disagreement with verbal content).

Sense of Self: In Schizophrenia there is a feeling of loss of individuality, identity, and self-direction. Ego boundaries are tenuous at best. Such individuals may appear perplexed as to who they are, and at the amount of control over their own destiny. This is especially prevalent if commanding delusions are present.

Volition: Ambivalence or lack of drive in the initiation and follow-up of goal-directed activities is usually present. As a result, there is gross impairment in overall functioning. This aspect of Schizophrenia is most readily observed in the Residual Phase of the disorder.

Impaired Interpersonal Functioning and Relationship to the External World: Fantasies and illogical, self-absorbed preoccupations cause the shutting out or distortion of the real world; withdrawal and emotional detachment are usually reported by significant others. At other times this impairment takes the form of exaggerated dependence, evidenced by excessive clinging, intrusiveness, and general failure to recognize another person's boundaries. This in turn elicits feelings of discomfort from others.

Psychomotor Behavior: Disturbances in this area, characterized by lack of appropriate reactivity to the environment, may take a variety of forms, from catatonic-like posturing, to extreme and purposeless motor movements.

DETERIORATION FROM HIGHEST LEVEL OF PREVIOUS FUNCTIONING

Schizophrenia always involves some form of deterioration from previous levels of functioning in such areas as school, work, self-care, and social relationships. These changes are usually reported by family members or those working closely with the individuals.

Prior to the onset of the Active Phase, which always involves psychotic symptoms, there may be a noticeable deterioration from previous functioning. This stage, called the Prodromal Phase, involves such symptoms as social withdrawal, disturbances of affect and communication, and regression in grooming and hygiene habits. At this time a change in personality becomes evident to those who know these individuals. Although the onset of this phase is difficult to determine, its length may be linked to the final outcome; the longer the Prodromal Phase, the worse the prognosis may be.

The Active Phase involves previously described disturbances of content and form of thought, perception, and affect. Usually the onset of this phase is brought about by a stressful life event. The psychotic symptoms in this phase must be present for at least 1 week unless there has been treatment with antipsychotic drugs.

After an Active Phase, return to the highest level of previous functioning is rare. Most commonly there is a Residual Phase which parallels the Prodromal Phase described above. If psychotic symptoms continue to be present, there is a decrease in their intensity.

DURATION

Duration of the illness is an important consideration in the diagnosis of Schizophrenia. There must be a continuous presence of symptoms for at least 6 months including those associated with the Active Phase.

TYPES OF SCHIZOPHRENIA

The *DSM-III-R* considers several types of Schizophrenia depending upon the predominant symptoms that precipitated the referral for evaluation. These types are: Disorganized, Catatonic, Paranoid, Undifferentiated, and Residual. Because the Catatonic and Paranoid types are extremely rare in children and adolescents, they are not included in this book.

Disorganized Type. The Disorganized Type's major presenting features are disturbances of affect and frequent incoherence, accompanied by fragmented delusions/hallucinations. Their lack of organization into systematized delusions/hallucinations is characteristic of this type of Schizophrenia.

Undifferentiated Type. The Undifferentiated Type presents delusions, hallucinations, incoherence, and disorganized behavior. However, none of these symptoms is particularly prominent upon referral, unlike other types of Schizophrenia.

Residual Type. The Residual Type requires a history of previous schizophrenic episodes, including the Active Phase. Although at the time of the evaluation, no psychotic symptoms are present, continuing evidence of the illness is manifested by affect disturbances, social withdrawal, oddities of behavior, and thought disturbances such as illogical or lack of cohesive speech.

(Consult Checklist on page 83.)

SCHIZOPHRENIA
INTERVIEW FORM

Active Phase Symptoms

    1. a. Does the person manifest delusionary thinking? Describe.

CHECKLIST

SCHIZOPHRENIA

Major Symptoms:

		Key
		+ Presence

-	Inattention
-	Impulsivity
+	Abnormal Activity Level
-	Aggressiveness
-	Violation of Rules
+	Isolation/Withdrawal/Avoidance
+	Inability to Form/Maintain Relationships
+	Disturbances of Affect or Mood
*	Anxiety
*	Depression
+	Delusions/Hallucinations
-	Somatic Complaints
+	Oddities of Behavior
+	Language Impairment
+	Impaired Cognition

Key

+ Presence

- Absence

* Associated Feature

Demographic Variables:

Age of Onset: Usually during adolescence or early adult-hood.

Duration: See text.

b. Are hallucinations present? If so, how often?

c. Is there incoherence, marked loosening of associations, poverty of speech content, or lack of logic in the individual's speech?

d. Is there a marked decrease in reactions to the environment, reduction in motor activity, mutism, or other forms of catatonic behavior?

e. Has the individual's affect shown significant changes from previous levels, such as blunting, flattening, or inappropriateness to the given situation?

2. Is delusionary thinking present and manifested by feelings of being controlled, thought broadcasting, thought insertion, or thought withdrawal?

3. Are auditory hallucinations reported in which either one voice critically comments on the individual's behavior, or two voices dialogue with each other?

4. Is there marked deterioration in the individual's overall functioning, such as at school, work, self-care, or in social relationships; or has there been failure to achieve the expected level of social development for his or her age?

5. How long have signs of the disturbance been present?

Prodromal or Residual Phase Symptoms

6. Have marked changes in social participation, such as withdrawal or isolation, been noted?

7. Has there been marked impairment in school or work performance?

8. Have strange behaviors on the part of the individual been reported, such as talking to self, hoarding food?

9. Have self-care and grooming habits deteriorated?

10. Has the individual's affect shown significant changes from previous levels, such as blunting, flattening, or inappropriateness to the given situation?

11. Does the individual's speech appear to be vague, stereotyped, metaphorical, or overly abstract or concrete?

12. Does the individual express bizarre ideas and beliefs, such as telepathic powers, clairvoyance, or superstitiousness?

13. Does the individual report that he or she is hearing, seeing, or sensing things which are not really there?
14. Does the individual show significant lack of initiative, interest, or energy?
15. Have organic factors for the presence of the previous symptoms been ruled out?

SCHIZOPHRENIA
CASE SUMMARY - Charles, C.A., 8-10

Psychiatric Summary: Charles was referred by his school for a multidisciplinary evaluation because of concerns about marked behavioral problems. He had previous evaluations beginning at 2 years of age, with various diagnoses leading to placement in several different educational programs.

As an infant, Charles stiffened when held and was difficult to console. At age 2, he began to have episodes of prolonged screaming, self-abuse, and sleeplessness. Currently he needs constant supervision for dressing, hygiene, eating, and safety. If unsupervised, he plays in the toilet, talks to himself, tries to climb walls, positions himself around the contours of furniture, and repeatedly plays with small cars. He continues to be attached to a pillow as a comfort item. In anxiety-producing situations, such as waiting at traffic lights, he tries to choke himself. Other concerns are for rare incontinence, frequent finger flicking, and hand flapping. He has no significant medical history.

On examination, Charles appeared healthy. He engaged in meaningless, repetitive play with objects while talking to himself. He made no direct eye contact, although he obviously attended peripherally. His responses to questions were very concrete. He verbalized many fears about monsters and required frequent reassurance regarding what was and was not real. Because of his very high degree of anxiety and flight of ideas, he was hospitalized and treated with major antipsychotic medication.

Psychological evaluation was difficult because of Charles' behavior, emotional lability, echolalia, and loose associations. Visual and auditory hallucinations were frequent, causing extreme anxiety. His language functioning was estimated below the 5th percentile. Educational assessment was difficult because of his behavior. Charles was functioning around the 1st grade level in both reading and math. Motor skills were also well below age level.

Following evaluation, Charles entered a pre-adolescent program at a psychiatric hospital for further treatment to decrease agitation and hallucinations. The diagnosis of Schizophrenia was made.

AUTHORS' COMMENTS

Charles exhibits many of the classic symptoms associated with Schizophrenia. His thought processes manifest loose associations and flight of ideas. Perceptual distortions involve auditory and visual hallucinations, including fears that overwhelm him. His impaired sense of self resulted in self-abusing behaviors; his relationship to the external world appears tenuous at best. Impaired psychomotor behavior took the form of purposeless motor movements such as finger flicking and other repetitive motions.

Deterioration in his level of functioning is demonstrated by extremely poor self-care habits, necessitating extraordinary supervision.

At first glance Charles appears to have a Pervasive Developmental Disorder. However, one of the primary differences between this disorder and Schizophrenia is the presence of the hallucinations and loosening associations reported in Charles' case.

ADDITIONAL READINGS
FOR SCHIZOPHRENIA

Achenbach, T. M. (1982). *Developmental Psychopathology* (2nd ed.). New York: John Wiley.

Cantor, S. (1988). *Childhood Schizophrenia.* New York: Guilford.

Schwartz, S., & Johnson, J. (1985). *Psychopathology of Childhood: A Clinical-Experimental Approach* (2nd ed.). New York: Pergamon.

Watt, N. F. (Ed.). (1984). *Children at Risk for Schizophrenia: A Longitudinal Perspective.* Cambridge: Cambridge University Press.

MAJOR DEPRESSIVE EPISODE

The diagnosis of Depression in children requires the occurrence of one or more Major Depressive Episodes. A

Major Depressive Episode may last from 2 weeks to 6 months and is primarily indicated by a depressed mood or loss of interest or pleasure.

The presence of depressed mood in children is usually inferred from the observations of others who know them, such as parents and teachers. They may report that these children look sad or unhappy, withdraw from social activities, or do not seem to care about previously enjoyed pursuits. Depressed children may also show disturbances of sleep patterns, such as sleeping too much or not enough. Appetite changes may be noted by either loss or gain of weight. Psychomotor disturbances could take the form of either increased agitation, such as inability to sit still, or decreased levels of energy, such as slowed body movements, poverty of speech, and complaints of fatigue. Difficulties in recall, concentration, and decision making are common, often negatively affecting school performance.

Some symptoms may not be readily observed and may require further probing. Among these are guilt, self-reproach, a sense of worthlessness, feelings of inadequacy, and harsh judgments of self. Other symptoms include anxiety, preoccupation with physical health, fears, and panic attacks. Suicidal ideation or thoughts of death may be present.

In children and adolescents, depression may be manifested by negativistic, aggressive behaviors, substance abuse, lack of cooperation at home and in school, poor hygiene, and restlessness. Particularly with adolescents, there is increased sensitivity to being criticized or rejected by others.

Major Depression involves all domains of the child's functioning. In the affective area there may be guilt, sadness, and tearfulness. In the cognitive area, there may be negative thinking about self and others. Motivation is affected by slowness of response or apathy. In the vegetative domain there are disturbances of sleep and eating patterns. Acting-out tendencies or decreased interaction with others are manifested in the social/behavioral domains.

DYSTHYMIA (or DEPRESSIVE NEUROSIS)

This disorder is considered chronic, lasting at least 1 year in children and adolescents. It is characterized by disturbances in mood such as depression and/or irritability.

This disorder can be manifested by such symptoms as disruptions in eating and sleeping patterns, low energy level, lack of self-worth, difficulties in concentration and attention, lack of goal-directed behavior, and feelings of hopelessness. Children with this disorder may have difficulties with social relationships, reacting shyly or angrily to peers and adults. School performance and occupational functioning may be adversely affected.

Dysthymia may co-exist with such disorders as Anorexia Nervosa and some Anxiety Disorders, but it is differentiated from Major Depression by its duration and severity. Because of its chronicity, children or adolescents with Dysthymia present a persistent pattern of impaired functioning. On the other hand, these children or adolescents may experience one or more distinct Major Depressive Episodes between times of their usual functioning.

(Consult Checklist on page 89.)

MAJOR DEPRESSIVE EPISODE/DYSTHYMIA INTERVIEW FORM

1. Has the child been unusually sad, unhappy, and tearful?
2. Has the child shown irritability, grouchiness, or low frustration tolerance?
3. Does the child seem unresponsive or apathetic towards previously enjoyed activities?
4. Has there been a change in his or her sleep patterns? Describe.
5. Has there been a change in his or her eating patterns? Describe, and indicate any fluctuation in weight.
6. Does the child seem overly active or unusually fatigued?
7. Has the child become oppositional, aggressive, and increasingly uncooperative?
8. Does the child show difficulties in concentration, attention to tasks, and decision-making skills?
9. Are there indicators of a sense of hopelessness and helplessness in the child?
10. Are there indicators of hypercritical judgments or guilt-ridden statements?

Clinical Evaluations of School-Aged Children

CHECKLIST

MAJOR DEPRESSIVE
EPISODE/DYSTHYMIA

Major Symptoms:

Key

*	Inattention
-	Impulsivity
*	Abnormal Activity Level
*	Aggressiveness
-	Violation of Rules
*	Isolation/Withdrawal/Avoidance
*	Inability to Form/Maintain Relationships
+	Disturbances of Affect or Mood
*	Anxiety
+	Depression
-	Delusions/Hallucinations
*	Somatic Complaints
-	Oddities of Behavior
-	Language Impairment
-	Impaired Cognition

Key:
+ Presence
- Absence
* Associated Feature

Demographic Variables:

Age of Onset: Usually begins in childhood, adolescence, or early adult life.
Duration: Major Depressive Episode - 2 weeks to 6 months.
Dysthymia - At least 1 year for children and adolescents.

89

11. Has the child become excessively fearful or avoidant of people or situations?
12. Has the child become overly preoccupied with his or her physical health?
13. Are there indicators of recurrent suicidal thoughts or gestures?
14. Is the child engaging in substance abuse? Describe.
15. Is the child described as withdrawn and isolated?
16. Have there been any changes in the child's personal hygiene habits?
17. Has school performance declined to a marked degree?

DYSTHYMIA
CASE SUMMARY - Larry, C.A., 11-0

Larry is an 11-year-old referred for an evaluation because of concern about his social skills, self-image, and acting-out behavior. He is in a small special education class because of moderate learning disabilities. The school reports that for at least 1-1/2 years, he has been increasingly distractible and easily frustrated. He frequently loses his temper and "sets himself up for rejection" by peers and adults. Larry dislikes team sports and is not involved in extra-curricular peer activities. He has difficulty falling asleep and has numerous somatic complaints.

Upon examination, Larry appeared depressed, with sad affect and much tearfulness. He was withdrawn and seemed extremely passive in his interactions with others. His interactions with peers have been increasingly conflicted, as he has instigated and provoked others. Larry is avoidant in discussing difficult issues and has trouble accepting responsibility for his actions. Personality testing suggests that he tends to externalize blame. His statements to the examiner indicated passivity, hopelessness, and lack of motivation to improve his relationships with peers and adults.

A recent intelligence test resulted in an average score with above-average performance on selected subtests. The psychologist noted that Larry's overall Average IQ may be a low estimate of his potential because of distractibility and lack of effort. Signs of depression were noted in his testing behavior as well as in the content of some of the responses.

In summary, Larry is a child of at least average intellectual potential who appears sad, anxious, has low self-esteem, and is easily overwhelmed by the social and emotional demands placed on him. A diagnosis of Dysthymia is made with recommendations for intensive therapeutic intervention for Larry and his family.

AUTHORS' COMMENTS

The chronicity of Larry's depressive symptoms justifies a diagnosis of Dysthymia. He presents many of the characteristics associated with this disorder, such as low self-esteem, irritability, sadness, poor social relationships, and marginal academic progress. Larry has been functioning within this general pattern for more than a year, precluding the existence of one or more discrete or specific Major Depressive Episodes.

ADDITIONAL READINGS
FOR DEPRESSION

Cicchetti, D., & Schneider-Rosen, K. (Eds.). (1984). *Childhood Depression.* San Francisco: Jossey-Bass.

Cytryn, L., & McKnew, D. (1979). Affective disorders. In J. Noshpitz (Ed.), *Basic Handbook of Child Psychiatry* (Vol. 2, pp. 321-340). New York: Basic Books.

French, A. P., & Berlin, I. N. (Eds.). (1979). *Depression in Children and Adolescents.* New York: Human Sciences Press.

Pfeffer, C. R. (1986). *The Suicidal Child.* New York: Guilford.

Rutter, M., & Izard, C. E. (Eds.). (1986). *Depression in Young People: Developmental and Clinical Perspectives.* New York: Guilford.

Trad, P. V. (1986). *Infant Depression: Paradigms and Paradoxes.* New York: Springer-Verlag.

Trad, P. V. (1987). *Infant and Childhood Depression: Developmental Factors.* New York: Wiley.

ELECTIVE MUTISM

There are no significant changes in the description of this disorder from the *DSM-III* to the revised edition.

Elective Mutism is characterized by a persistent refusal to speak in social situations, including school, in spite of usually intact language skills. There may be some articulation and/or language delays in a small number of these children.

Children with this disorder attempt communication by nonverbal gesturing or monosyllabic utterances. They are often described as very shy, clinging, and socially withdrawn in unfamiliar situations. They often refuse to go to school. In the home they may be oppositional, demanding, and prone to temper tantrums. Often these children suffer from emotional badgering by their peers. Impairment in social and school functioning is likely to occur because of their reluctance to communicate and participate.

Factors that may precipitate this disorder include early traumatic experiences, parental overprotection, immigration to a country with a different language, and abnormal speech or cognitive development.

(Consult Checklist on page 93.)

ELECTIVE MUTISM
INTERVIEW FORM

1. Does the child have the ability to speak and comprehend language? If yes,
2. Does he or she persistently refuse to speak in most social situations, including school?
3. How does he or she communicate?
4. Does the child show any of the following?

   a. excessive shyness
   b. clinging
   c. social withdrawal
   d. school refusal
   e. oppositional behaviors

5. Describe the child's school functioning, socially and academically.
6. Has the child been diagnosed as having a speech disorder?
7. Has the child been exposed to a physical or emotional trauma? Explain.
8. Explore the degree of independence fostered in the child by his or her parents.
9. Has the family recently immigrated to a country where another language is spoken?

CHECKLIST

ELECTIVE MUTISM

Major Symptoms:

Key

-	Inattention
-	Impulsivity
-	Abnormal Activity Level
*	Aggressiveness
-	Violation of Rules
+	Isolation/Withdrawal/Avoidance
+	Inability to Form/Maintain Relationships
-	Disturbances of Affect or Mood
*	Anxiety
*	Depression
-	Delusions/Hallucinations
-	Somatic Complaints
+	Oddities of Behavior
*	Language Impairment
-	Impaired Cognition

Key:
+ Presence
- Absence
* Associated Feature

Demographic Variables:

Age of Onset: Usually before age 5.
Duration: Variable from a few weeks to several years.

ELECTIVE MUTISM
CASE SUMMARY - Thomas, C.A., 7-3

Clinical Summary: Thomas was referred for a complete evaluation because of his refusal to speak at school. This problem became apparent when he started nursery school at age 3. He would not speak to other students or teachers. He spent his school day sitting apart from the group and watching. At home he spoke with his family and would speak to other children outside of school. With a lot of encouragement he had started to speak in a whisper to his teacher, and to speak to other children on the playground. However, other children tended to ignore him and he has seemed "odder" as he has gotten older. One year ago he was referred to a psychiatric clinic and a behavior management program was begun to facilitate eye contact and interaction. Because of lack of progress, the current evaluation was requested.

There was no significant medical history other than several ear infections. He had tubes inserted twice but currently has normal hearing. The parents felt that his receptive and expressive language skills were normal. They felt that he was not affectionate and was possibly depressed.

The family consisted of mother and father, both high-school graduates, Thomas, and a 5-year-old sibling who had also been very quiet upon entering school.

On examination, the boy made little eye contact, keeping a baseball cap pulled down over his forehead at all times. He responded to instructions but said nothing. During evaluation sessions, Thomas' mother requested that she be allowed to sit outside the examiner's room. Thomas performed above his 2nd grade level in all academic tasks but would not verbalize. A speech and language evaluation was accomplished by the mother administering the test items. His receptive and expressive language skills were normal.

Intellectual assessment indicated average results. Personality assessment indicated an array of ego deficits, including strong dependency needs, strong feelings of insecurity, and lack of trust. His control over his own verbalizations was felt to represent his attempt to exert control over his life in one of the few ways he could. All evaluators agreed on a diagnosis of Elective Mutism. Recommendation was made for a psychiatrically based day treatment program.

AUTHORS' COMMENTS

Although Thomas understands language and can speak, he has persistently refused to do so in school. He has exhibited such behaviors for the past 4 years. From the descriptions of his symptoms, he presents himself as an overly dependent youngster who would only perform the required tasks in his mother's presence. As stated by the psychiatrist, Thomas' refusal to speak suggests an attempt to exert control over some aspect of his life.

Thomas demonstrated some of the additional features associated with this disorder. He was generally oppositional during the examination, refusing to cooperate with many of the doctor's requests. Social withdrawal and inability to initiate peer interaction were also noted.

These behaviors meet the diagnostic criteria for Elective Mutism. The recommendation for a day treatment program illustrates the extent and severity of his disorder.

ADDITIONAL READINGS
FOR ELECTIVE MUTISM

Laybourne, P. (1979). Elective mutism. In J. Noshpitz (Ed.), *Basic Handbook of Child Psychiatry* (Vol. 2, pp. 475-481). New York: Basic Books.

Nash, R. T., Thorpe, H. W., & Andrews, M. (1979). A management program for elective mutism. *Psychology in the Schools, 16*, 246-252.

Schakel, J. A. (1983). The treatment of elective mutism in children within the school setting: Two case studies. *School Psychology Review, 12*, 467-471

INTRODUCTION

This class of disorders includes Gender Identity Disorder of Childhood, Transsexualism, Gender Identity Disorder of Adolescence or Adulthood-Nontranssexual Type (GIDAANT), and Gender Identity Disorder Not Otherwise Specified.

The essential feature of all these disorders is the disparity between the physical sexual characteristics of the individuals and their knowledge and awareness of their particular gender. Disturbances in gender identity range from mild to severe ambiguity about one's sex assignment. In mild cases there is awareness, yet discomfort about the assigned sex. In severe cases, such as Transsexualism, there is a strong sense of not belonging to one's assigned sex but instead, to the opposite one. This book will only address Gender Identity Disorder of Childhood.

GENDER IDENTITY DISORDER OF CHILDHOOD

For both sexes, this disorder is manifested by feelings of extreme uneasiness, rejection of their own physical sex attributes, and strong proclivity to be of the other sex. This disorder is differentiated from the usual tomboyish or sissy-like behaviors, by the significant degree of these children's rejection of their own sex assignment and identification with the opposite one.

For boys there is intense interest in feminine clothing, traditional feminine activities such as playing house, playing with dolls, and dressing up in women's clothing, and a desire to be included in groups of girls. Boys with this disorder avoid masculine groups, interests, and activities such as sports and rough outdoor playing. Aside from feminine pursuits, there is a strong and pervasive denial of their physical sex characteristics and a wish that these would disappear.

For girls there is interest in masculine activities, groups, sports, and rough-and-tumble play. There is avoidance of participation in female groups and culturally expected feminine activities. There is also a strong and pervasive denial of their physical sex characteristics and a wish that these would disappear. Girls may state that they are biologically unable to bear children.

This disorder can manifest itself as early as 4 years of age, resulting in overt social conflict by the time the child is 7 or 8 years old.

In boys with this disorder there may be extreme physical and emotional attachment to the mother and relative distance from or passivity towards the father figure. In girls there may be a history of maternal unavailability because of neglect or abandonment, forcing overidentification with the father.

Social impairment for both sexes is significant both at home and in school. These children tend to be isolated, ostracized, and teased by others, especially by those of their same-sex peer group. This may result in a refusal to attend school.

CHECKLIST

GENDER IDENTITY
DISORDER OF CHILDHOOD

Major Symptoms:

Key

+	Presence
-	Absence
*	Associated Feature

- Inattention

- Impulsivity

- Abnormal Activity Level

- Aggressiveness

- Violation of Rules

* Isolation/Withdrawal/Avoidance

* Inability to Form/Maintain Relationships

- Disturbances of Affect or Mood

* Anxiety

* Depression

- Delusions/Hallucinations

- Somatic Complaints

+ Oddities of Behavior

- Language Impairment

- Impaired Cognition

Demographic Variables:

Age of Onset: By age 7.
Duration: Unspecified.

GENDER IDENTITY
DISORDER OF CHILDHOOD
INTERVIEW FORM

For Females:

1. Does the girl state a strong desire to be a boy, or insist that she is a boy?
2. Does the girl persistently negate feminine anatomical features as evidenced by any of the following?

    a. Asserts that she has or will grow a penis.
    b. Refuses to urinate in a sitting position.
    c. Asserts that she does not want to grow breasts or menstruate.

3. Does the girl persistently refuse to wear feminine clothing and insist upon wearing typically masculine clothing instead?
4. Has the girl reached puberty?
5. Does she avoid participating in activities with same-sex groups?
6. Describe her play activities, interests, and choice of toys.
7. Has a female figure been unavailable in the home?
8. Describe how friends and family members react to the girl's tendencies towards masculine activity.
9. Has there been refusal to attend school?

For Males:

1. Does the boy state a strong desire to be a girl, or insist that he is a girl?
2. Does the boy persistently negate male anatomical features as evidenced by any of the following?

    a. That he will grow up to become a woman.
    b. That his penis or testes are repugnant or will disappear.
    c. That it would be better not to have a penis or testes.

3. Is he overly preoccupied with female activities, such as cross-dressing or participation in girls' games?
4. Has the boy reached puberty?

5. Does he avoid participating in activities with same-sex groups?
6. Describe his play activities, interests, and choice of toys.
7. Has a male figure been unavailable at home?
8. Describe how friends and family members react to the child's tendencies towards feminine activity.
9. Has there been refusal to attend school?

GENDER IDENTITY
DISORDER OF CHILDHOOD
CASE SUMMARY - Mark, C.A., 11-0

Mark was referred for evaluation because of excessive absenteeism from school. His parents were divorced when he was 6 months old, with no subsequent contacts by his father. He is kept at home by his mother whenever he has a headache, which occurs several days per week. On the rare days that he does go to school, he is apt to go to the school nurse complaining of a headache. Mark usually remains at home by himself or accompanies his mother to her job. He participates in no peer group activities but enjoys fishing, which he does alone. His only close friend of the same age is his female cousin who lives next door.

During the evaluation the examiner was quite impressed with several behaviors which made her feel uncomfortable. Mark would brush his hair away from his face and angle his cheek towards the examiner prior to making a verbal response. He had elaborate hand gestures which had a feminine quality to them. Mark also showed unusual interest in the examiner's clothes and asked where she had purchased them.

During the clinical interview, Mark stated wishes to be a girl, explaining that he felt more comfortable participating in activities such as dressing up in his mother's clothing when she was not home. He also disclosed that he has a collection of dolls, which he keeps hidden in his closet and with which he only plays when alone or with his cousin. Mark's human figure drawing was a detailed rendering of a female. He refused to draw a male when requested to do so.

Mark stated that he was constantly teased by peers in school because he did not want to participate in any sports or group activities with the other boys, and because

99

he preferred to stay with the girls during recess and at lunch.

Upon psychiatric examination, the diagnosis of Gender Identity Disorder of Childhood was made.

AUTHORS' COMMENTS

It is not clear from the clinical interview the extent of Mark's discomfort with his own male anatomical features, but his refusal to draw a male figure suggests discomfort associated with his gender identity. This seems to be supported by his significant interest in female characteristics. Mark's behavior associated with this disorder has caused isolation from his peer group and school refusal.

ADDITIONAL READINGS FOR GENDER IDENTITY DISORDER OF CHILDHOOD

Green, R. (1974). *Sexual Identity Conflict in Children and Adults.* New York: Basic Books.

Money, J., & Erhardt, A. A. (1972). *Man and Woman, Boy and Girl: Differentiation and Dimorphism of Gender Identity from Conception to Maturity.* Baltimore: Johns Hopkins University Press.

IDENTITY DISORDER

There are no major changes in the description of this disorder from the *DSM-III* to its revised edition.

Identity disorder is characterized by prolonged uncertainty accompanied by severe discomfort, anxiety, and depression about long-term goals associated with lifestyles, career choices, and moral value systems.

Individuals with this disorder lack a realistic appraisal of themselves; they have difficulty making decisions about major aspects of their lives or they make impulsive choices, resulting in frequent changes in jobs, careers, and relationships. These conflicts usually result in varied degrees of impairment related to academic, social, and occupational functioning.

Because these individuals seek a definition of their identity, assumption of a wide variety of contrasting roles is not uncommon. Some of these may involve purposefully divergent values from those expected by the family, straining familial ties.

If this disorder persists over time, individuals may be severely impaired in their ability to establish long-term emotional bonds and dedication to occupational pursuits. The severity of stress and impairment in social and academic functioning differentiates this disorder from the usual adolescent dilemmas about identity. If a pervasive pattern of instability affecting mood, self-image, and interpersonal relationships continues after age 18, and becomes more entrenched in the personality, then a diagnosis of Borderline Personality Disorder is made.

(Consult Checklist on page 102.)

IDENTITY DISORDER
INTERVIEW FORM

1. Does the adolescent express severe worry, heightened anxiety, or indecision about any of the following?

   a. long-term goals
   b. career choices
   c. friendship patterns
   d. sexual orientation and behavior
   e. religious identification
   f. moral value systems
   g. group loyalties

2. Does this distress affect school, work, or social functioning? Describe.
3. How long has this distress persisted?
4. Has the individual experimented with a variety of roles, such as cults, religious affiliations, group associations, or multiple occupational fields?
5. How long is he or she able to maintain a commitment to any of his or her choices?
6. Does the individual seek definition of self by asking or implying lack of knowledge of his or her own identity, such as by asking, "Who am I"?
7. How congruent are his or her life choices with the values of his or her family?

IDENTITY DISORDER
CASE SUMMARY - Robert, C.A., 14-0

Reason for Referral: Robert was referred for psychiatric evaluation because of increasing oppositional and

CHECKLIST

IDENTITY DISORDER

Major Symptoms:

<table>
<tr><td></td><td></td><td>Key</td></tr>
</table>

		Key
-	Inattention	+ Presence
-	Impulsivity	- Absence
-	Abnormal Activity Level	* Associated Feature
-	Aggressiveness	
-	Violation of Rules	
-	Isolation/Withdrawal/Avoidance	
+	Inability to Form/Maintain Relationships	
*	Disturbances of Affect or Mood	
+	Anxiety	
+	Depression	
-	Delusions/Hallucinations	
-	Somatic Complaints	
-	Oddities of Behavior	
-	Language Impairment	
-	Impaired Cognition	

Demographic Variables:

Age of Onset: Late adolescence, before age 18.
Duration: At least 3 months.

negative behaviors at home and school. His school performance had been dropping for at least the past year, and he displayed characteristics of depression and withdrawal. At school Robert was reportedly verbally abusive, displayed poor impulse control, was attention seeking, had problems in his peer relationships, demonstrated a high activity level, and had difficulty deferring gratification. In addition there were some concerns expressed about his sexual orientation, reportedly manifested by unisex clothing, jewelry, and effeminate body gestures. These behaviors have reportedly caused significant distress and conflict among family members.

Observations: Robert entered the interview room readily and without hesitance. He was flamboyant in his manner and bizarrely dressed. He wore a white headband tied so as to push his hair up in a pompadour style. Robert wore a white t-shirt with a black vest, black sunglasses worn on a cord around his neck, black sneakers with white shoelaces, a studded leather wristlet, and studded belt with a large buckle bearing a red heart and initials. Robert had long black hair, very long artificial fingernails on his fourth and fifth fingers, and small black cords simulating rings on his ring finger. He displayed some effeminate characteristics and was quite self-centered and dramatic in his posturing throughout the interview.

Interview: As we discussed behavior that related to sexual orientation, Robert became somewhat vague and tangential. He reported that many girls have liked him but that he "must think of myself"; consequently he must be selective in his choices. He was angry about comments regarding his hanging around with older kids and working in a massage parlor. He added that he went there specifically to see two girls but that he only knocks on the door and talks with them. Asked about homosexual feelings or fantasies, Robert alluded to experiencing homosexual feelings only once and did not wish to discuss it further.

Robert said that he gets along fine with other kids unless they are "playing with my mind." He then slaps them down either verbally or physically.

In his fantasy materials Robert had rather omnipotent and grandiose dreams of fame, wealth, and stardom. He dreamt of utilizing his singing talent professionally and of pursuing vocational goals at the technical school where he hopes to learn about shop and hairdressing. He spoke about a wide variety of other interests and ambitions for the future, including college attendance, studying political science, microbiology, or computer science.

Summary: This 14-year-old, 8th-grade student displays many characteristics of a highly ambivalent sexual orientation. He is effeminate in many of his mannerisms, engages in cross-gender dress, and strongly identifies with female traits and characteristics. However, he himself describes a heterosexual orientation in his ideation, fantasy life, and behavior. His homosexual fantasies are at a minimum. Since Robert is highly exhibitionistic and dramatic in his style, one must assume that there is at least a mixed sexual orientation at the present time. The fact that he uses his homosexual orientation characteristics as an attention-getting device leads this evaluator to conclude that one cannot be sure how much Robert is motivated by an orientation preference, and how much he is motivated by the need to generate shock in those around him.

Highly manipulative, Robert is likely to attempt to maneuver adults into allowing him to get his own way. This is certainly consistent with his high level of egocentrism and demanding nature. Socially, it is probable that Robert enjoys his association with the fringe element in the community because it gives him a sense of status and excitement.

Diagnosis: Identity Disorder.

AUTHORS' COMMENTS

Robert shows significant indecision about his sexual orientation and behavior, friendship patterns, career choices, and long-term goals. His dress and demeanor tend to be effeminate; he is beginning to associate with undesirable companions; and he has several unrealistic, grandiose dreams of fame, wealth, and stardom. In reality, Robert's school functioning has declined considerably during the past year. His present choices are distressing to the members of his family and further impair his social functioning.

The *DSM-III-R* particularly emphasizes the distress and anxiety involved in lack of resolution regarding such choices. Robert's level of distress has not been explored in the current report, although withdrawal and depression were noted in his referral.

ADDITIONAL READINGS
FOR IDENTITY DISORDER

Erikson, E. H. (1968). *Identity, Youth, and Crisis.* New York: Norton.
Levine, S., Korenblum, M., & Golombek, H. (1983). Disorders commonly appearing first during adolescence. In P. Steinhauer & Q. Rae-Grant (Eds.), *Psychological Problems of the Child in the Family* (pp. 414-416). New York: Basic Books.
Rutter, M., Graham, P., & Chadwick, O. (1976). Adolescent turmoil-fact or fiction? *Journal of Child Psychology and Psychiatry, 17,* 35-76.

REACTIVE ATTACHMENT DISORDER
OF INFANCY AND EARLY CHILDHOOD

In the *DSM-III*, this disorder pertained exclusively to infants, before the age of 8 months. It was mostly characterized by failure to thrive, lack of social responsivity, and limited physical development. These symptoms were attributed to poor caretaking with respect to physical and emotional needs.

The *DSM-III-R* has expanded criteria for this disorder to include early childhood, up to the age of 5 years. It is characterized by marked disturbance in social relatedness. Children with this disorder may manifest persistent lack of initiative or response in social situations, such as absence of visual contact or social initiative, and lack of cooperative play and spontaneity. These children may also be excessively familiar with strangers, showing indiscriminate affection.

In infants, this disorder is manifested mostly by lack of attention, interest, or visual or vocal interaction with the caretaker. There is indifference to being held or picked up; no facial expression indicating joy, surprise, fear, or anger. These children may have poor muscle tone, a weak cry, sleep excessively, have feeding disturbances, and show a general lack of interest in the environment. They are initially brought to the attention of the physician because of their physical failure to grow, or because of another physical complication.

To obtain a diagnosis of Reactive Attachment Disorder of Infancy and Early Childhood, a thorough investigation of the quality of care, both physical and emotional, must be undertaken. Such children may have been abused or neglected, may have had several different caretakers, may have been exposed to physical danger, and likely did not receive attention to their basic emotional needs.

Their caregivers may be experiencing significant depression, may lack support from important others, may have disturbances of impulse control, and/or may have been victims of abuse or neglect in childhood. Other factors may include long periods of separation after birth, either because of an infant's placement in an incubator, or inability to secure a home for an adoptable child. Further confirmation of the diagnosis of Reactive Attachment Disorder of Infancy and Early Childhood is made by the recovery observed in such children once they are given adequate care and attention.

(Consult Checklist on page 107.)

REACTIVE ATTACHMENT DISORDER
OF INFANCY AND EARLY CHILDHOOD
INTERVIEW FORM

1. Describe the child's social relatedness to others.
2. Describe the child's physical condition.
3. Has a physical examination of the child been conducted recently?
4. How long has the caretaker been known to the child?
5. Describe the quality of the relationship between the child and the caretaker.
6. Does the child convey emotions through facial expressions?
7. Does the child initiate and/or respond to play activities?
8. Does the child show normal alertness, curiosity, and interest in his or her environment?
9. Does the child show disturbances in eating or sleeping patterns?
10. Is there evidence of physical abuse, or emotional or physical neglect?

CHECKLIST

REACTIVE ATTACHMENT DISORDER
OF INFANCY AND EARLY CHILDHOOD

Major Symptoms:

Key

+	Inattention
-	Impulsivity
+	Abnormal Activity Level
-	Aggressiveness
-	Violation of Rules
+	Isolation/Withdrawal/Avoidance
+	Inability to Form/Maintain Relationships
-	Disturbances of Affect or Mood
-	Anxiety
-	Depression
-	Delusions/Hallucinations
+	Somatic Complaints
-	Oddities of Behavior
*	Language Impairment
-	Impaired Cognition

Key

+ Presence

- Absence

* Associated
  Feature

Demographic Variables:

Age of Onset: Before 5 years.
Duration: Unspecified.

107

REACTIVE ATTACHMENT DISORDER
OF INFANCY AND EARLY CHILDHOOD
CASE SUMMARY - Peter, C.A., 3-2

Peter was brought to the attention of the pediatrician by a neighbor who was concerned at seeing the boy unattended for a long period of time.

Upon examination, the child was found to be grossly underweight, unresponsive, and physically neglected. His cry was noted to be weak, with overall poor motility. Peter seemed apathetic and unwilling or unable to respond verbally to the pediatrician. He did not explore any toys available in the office.

Further investigation revealed a young single mother with no family support in the area. She was depressed, and felt lonely and unable to care for her child, whom she described as "difficult to handle." She, herself, had been adopted after spending most of her early childhood in several different foster placements.

Peter was hospitalized to treat his failure to thrive. A social worker met with the mother and convinced her to join a parenting group. Within a month Peter physically began to thrive; he also showed increasing alertness and social interest. Both Peter and his mother are being monitored by a social agency.

A diagnosis of Reactive Attachment Disorder of Infancy and Early Childhood was made.

AUTHORS' COMMENTS

Peter shows many of the symptoms associated with this disorder. He appeared uncommunicative, and was obviously underweight and neglected. His physical and emotional needs were not being met by a mother who was alone, depressed, and frustrated with her son's normal childhood demands. She did not appear equipped to care adequately for the child, as she herself had been the victim of an unstable environment. The results of the therapeutic intervention designed for Peter and his mother further confirmed the appropriateness of the diagnosis.

EATING DISORDERS

INTRODUCTION

These disorders are characterized by significant disturbances in eating patterns. Anorexia Nervosa and Rumination Disorder of Infancy may be life threatening. Pica and Rumination Disorder of Infancy are primarily found in young children, while the onset of Anorexia Nervosa and Bulimia Nervosa is typically in adolescence or early adulthood.

Changes in criteria from the *DSM-III* to the *DSM-III-R* include percentage of weight loss in Anorexia Nervosa (25% to 15%) and the inclusion of disruption in the menstrual cycle for females as one of the symptoms of this disorder. In Bulimia Nervosa, consideration is given to the number of binge episodes per week and preoccupation with body shape and weight. While still common in Bulimia Nervosa, the following behaviors have been excluded from the specific criteria for diagnosis: types of food ingested, weight fluctuation, secretive eating, and depression following binges. The diagnostic criteria for Pica and Rumination Disorder of Infancy have essentially remained unchanged in the *DSM-III-R*.

ANOREXIA NERVOSA

This disorder cannot be attributed to a physical condition and does not initially involve loss of appetite. Anorexia Nervosa focuses on severe body image distortion, intense fear of becoming obese, and amenorrhea in females, with significant weight loss and refusal to maintain at least normal body weight.

These individuals show a marked preoccupation with body size, scrutinizing themselves in an obsessive manner. Fear of obesity results in reduction of food intake, self-induced vomiting, use of laxatives, and prolonged physical exercise. When unable to control food intake, behaviors associated with Bulimia Nervosa may be present, such as food binging and vomiting.

Diagnosis of Anorexia Nervosa is considered when at least 15% of the original body weight is lost and/or a minimal relationship between height and weight is not maintained.

Physical signs of Anorexia may include edema, hypotension, and hypothermia. Marked decrease in or lack of psychosexual development and compulsive habits are often present. Denial and resistance to therapy are not uncommon, and in most cases hospitalization is the usual course of treatment.

Individuals suffering from this disorder tend to be described as overly perfectionistic, "ideal children." About 34% are reported to be slightly overweight before the onset of the illness. Females represent 95% of the reported cases of Anorexia Nervosa. In many instances a stressful episode may trigger this disorder.

(Consult Checklist on page 113.)

ANOREXIA NERVOSA
INTERVIEW FORM

1. Does the person express intense fear of being obese in contrast to his or her actual body weight?
2. Does the person complain of feeling fat while his or her weight is normal?
3. Does the person refuse to maintain minimal body weight for age and height?
4. How much weight has the person lost?
5. In females, has there been any disruption in menstrual cycles?
6. Does the person acknowledge or realize that his or her behavior is abnormal?
7. Does the person engage in excessive use of laxatives, or self-induced vomiting?
8. Is the person preoccupied with his or her body image; for instance, frequently staring at the mirror, stating dissatisfaction with specific body parts?
9. Describe any unusual behaviors associated with food, such as limiting intake to low-caloric foods, binge eating, hoarding, concealment, and throwing food away?
10. Has there been a recent stressful event in the person's life?
11. Has a recent medical examination ruled out physical causes for the weight loss?

CHECKLIST

ANOREXIA NERVOSA

Major Symptoms:

-	Inattention
-	Impulsivity
-	Abnormal Activity Level
-	Aggressiveness
-	Violation of Rules
*	Isolation/Withdrawal/Avoidance
-	Inability to Form/Maintain Relationships
-	Disturbances of Affect or Mood
-	Anxiety
-	Depression
-	Delusions/Hallucinations
+	Somatic Complaints
+	Oddities of Behavior
-	Language Impairment
-	Impaired Cognition

Key

+ Presence
- Absence
* Associated Feature

Demographic Variables:

Age of Onset: Early to late adolescence.
Duration: Weight loss of at least 15% of original body weight.

113

12. Does the person engage in obsessive/compulsive behaviors such as frequent hand washing?

ANOREXIA NERVOSA
CASE SUMMARY - Nadia, C.A., 12-4

Nadia, a 12-year-old girl, was referred for hospitalization by her pediatrician because of a 17-pound weight loss over the past 3 months. She denied vomiting and diarrhea but had complained in the past of constipation. She had reduced her food and liquid intake markedly, which caused significant family stress. The family then forced her to eat. In spite of having dropped from the 50th to the 5th percentile in weight (for height), Nadia felt she was of normal weight. She was an honor student and an immaculate housekeeper. All her friends are achievers, but she had recently become socially withdrawn. She is not and never has been very communicative with her parents.

Her past medical history was unremarkable. The family consists of her parents, both high school graduates, and their two daughters, Nadia being the older. A new baby was expected in 2 months.

Nadia was begun on bed rest, with increasing privileges in response to weight gain. Calorie counts were maintained. She was seen for daily psychotherapy while an inpatient. It was felt that her eating disorder was the response to the stresses of impending adolescence, coupled with the anticipated changes in her family constellation by the birth of a new, much younger sibling. Nadia was hospitalized for 6 weeks, then discharged to continue outpatient therapy. Although she continued to be overly preoccupied with food intake, she was able to maintain approximate weight.

AUTHORS' COMMENTS

Nadia had lost more than 15% of her body weight for her size, which could not be accounted for by any medical condition. She significantly reduced her own food intake while denying that she was losing weight. Attempts by the family to force food intake probably created more stress for her.

Children with this disorder are often described as high achievers and meticulous to the point of being compulsive. Another commonly found feature involves withdrawal from peer group activities, which was apparent in Nadia's case.

Anorexia Nervosa may be precipitated by a stressor; in Nadia's case, the onset of adolescence as well as the birth of a new sibling were the stressors identified by the psychologist.

BULIMIA NERVOSA

In this disorder there is acknowledgement of abnormal eating patterns accompanied by depression, self-punishing statements or thoughts after binging, and fear of not being able to control eating. The person's life appears to be dominated by conflicts about eating.

Binge eating may be planned and involves the rapid consumption of large amounts of food, usually chosen for their sweet taste, high caloric content, and form which enables fast eating. Consumption is done secretly with limited chewing, to consume as much food as possible in the shortest amount of time. Sleep, induced vomiting, stomach pain, or interruption by others usually ends a binge. Vomiting usually follows a binge because it relieves abdominal pain, reduces anxiety, and allows for either continuation or termination of a binge.

For a diagnosis of Bulimia Nervosa, individuals must engage in an average of two binge episodes a week for at least 3 months. Fluctuation of weight is common but not life threatening; some individuals appear under- or overweight as a result of recurrent episodes of binging and fasting. There is uncommon preoccupation with body appearance and frequent attempts at controlling weight gain by strict dieting, fasting, use of laxatives or diuretics, or vigorous exercise. Abuse of other substances, such as barbiturates, amphetamines, cocaine, or alcohol, may be present.

(Consult Checklist on page 116.)

BULIMIA NERVOSA
INTERVIEW FORM

1. Does the person engage in recurrent binge eating?
2. Is the person aware that his or her eating pattern is abnormal and is he or she fearful of not being able to control it?

CHECKLIST
BULIMIA NERVOSA

Major Symptoms:

Key

-	Inattention
-	Impulsivity
-	Abnormal Activity Level
-	Aggressiveness
-	Violation of Rules
-	Isolation/Withdrawal/Avoidance
-	Inability to Form/Maintain Relationships
*	Disturbances of Affect or Mood
*	Anxiety
*	Depression
-	Delusions/Hallucinations
*	Somatic Complaints
+	Oddities of Behavior
-	Language Impairment
-	Impaired Cognition

Key

+ Presence

- Absence

* Associated Feature

Demographic Variables:

Age of Onset: Adolescence.
Duration: Minimum average of two binge episodes per week for at least 3 months.

116

3. Is there excessive use of laxatives, self-induced vomiting, use of diuretics, severely restrictive diets, or strenuous exercise in attempts to lose weight?
4. Is the person overly preoccupied with his or her body image?
5. How often does the person engage in binging episodes?
6. Is the binging behavior characterized by any of the following?

   a. Consumption of high-caloric, easily ingested foods.
   b. Inconspicuous or secretive eating during a binge.
   c. Termination of such eating episodes by sleep, abdominal pain, self-induced vomiting, or social interruption.

7. Does the person appear depressed and/or express self-punishing thoughts following binge eating?
8. Does he or she engage in abuse of substances such as alcohol, cocaine, sedatives, or amphetamines?

BULIMIA NERVOSA
CASE SUMMARY - Debbie, C.A., 16-2

Debbie was initially seen by the school nurse, who referred her for further evaluation to a nearby clinic.

Medical Findings: Debbie is a high school sophomore who was referred for medical care because of pain and swelling of the left side of her face. Detailed history was obtained. She had been overweight 4 years earlier and, under medical supervision, lost 24 pounds. She was now at approximately her ideal body weight. However, maintaining her weight was difficult. Debbie was very involved in exercise and used it for weight maintenance.

One and a half years ago at Christmas, she began vomiting after large meals. The vomiting became more frequent and when she came in for evaluation, she was vomiting almost every day after meals. At first she denied the use of laxatives, emetics, diet pills, and diuretics, but later admitted using laxatives and self-induced vomiting to control her weight.

Upon inquiry on her eating patterns, Debbie stated that she tends to ingest large quantities of food secretly, especially pizzas, cakes, and cookies. Following a binge, Debbie attempts to fast for several days. She expressed anger with herself for not being able to control these urges and admitted being overly preoccupied with food.

On physical examination, Debbie had swelling and tenderness of the left parotid, a salivary gland. She was pale and appeared unhealthy. She lacked energy. Her lab work revealed iron deficiency anemia. She was hospitalized to stabilize her medical condition and to begin family-oriented therapy. A diagnosis of Bulimia Nervosa was made.

AUTHORS' COMMENTS

This case clearly illustrates the binge and purge pattern of eating present in Bulimia Nervosa, the psychological factors associated with it, and some of the physical consequences of this disorder.

PICA

This disorder is characterized by the intake of non-food substances when there is no aversion present to common foods. Infants usually ingest paint, plaster, hair, cloth, or string. Older children may eat bugs, sand, leaves, droppings, or stones. The most common physical complications of this disorder are lead poisoning, associated with paint intake, and intestinal obstructions as a result of ingestion of foreign objects. Deficiencies in certain minerals (iron, zinc), poor parental supervision, and mental retardation may be associated with this disorder.

(Consult Checklist on page 119.)

PICA
INTERVIEW FORM

1. Does the child engage in persistent eating of non-food substances? Describe.
2. For how long has the pattern of eating been observed?
3. Is he or she interested in consuming appropriate food substances?

118

CHECKLIST

PICA

Major Symptoms:

Key

-	Inattention
-	Impulsivity
-	Abnormal Activity Level
-	Aggressiveness
-	Violation of Rules
-	Isolation/Withdrawal/Avoidance
-	Inability to Form/Maintain Relationships
-	Disturbances of Affect or Mood
-	Anxiety
-	Depression
-	Delusions/Hallucinations
-	Somatic Complaints
+	Oddities of Behavior
-	Language Impairment
*	Impaired Cognition

Key
+ Presence
- Absence
* Associated Feature

Demographic Variables:

Age of Onset: Usually between 12 and 24 months.
Duration: At least 1 month.

4. If consumption of paint has occurred, has the child been examined recently by a physician for lead poisoning?
5. Is there adequate supervision at home?

PICA
CASE SUMMARY -
Beth, C.A., 6-3; Susan, C.A., 4-5

A medical report was received by the school as a result of developmental assessments and follow-up for both girls.

Beth and Susan are half-sisters who are being followed medically because of their past history of lead poisoning. An initial diagnosis of lead poisoning was made on the basis of routine blood screening when Beth was 2-1/2 years and Susan was 6 months old. At the time the blood was tested, Beth was irritable and had a decreased appetite, and Susan was failing to thrive.

The children lived with their mother in an older, multifamily house, which had a high lead level in the paint on the bathroom walls and on the windowsills throughout. Both children were noted to pick up nonfood items and mouth them.

The children were admitted to the hospital for therapy on three occasions over 7 months. Only after the third admission were they finally moved to lead-free housing. Current developmental assessment indicated significant concerns about their language development, distractibility, and attention span, with recommendations for special school placement.

AUTHORS' COMMENTS

This case illustrates a long-term pattern of eating nonfood substances containing lead, and the harmful consequences of such behaviors both physically and cognitively.

RUMINATION DISORDER OF INFANCY

Infants with this disorder convey the impression of considerable pleasure from repeated regurgitation of partially digested food. Usually the food is released from the mouth or chewed and swallowed again. Nausea, gastrointestinal pain, and rejection of food do not accompany this disorder. Its onset occurs after a period of normal food intake. Between episodes of throwing up, the infant may display signs of irritability, usually associated with hunger.

This disorder can be life threatening because of weight loss or malnutrition. As a result of the infant's behavior, the primary caretaker may feel discouraged in the attempts to feed the baby and may become passive, avoid the child, and refrain from normal stimulation. If not successfully treated, delays in all aspects of the child's development may occur.

(Consult Checklist on page 122.)

RUMINATION DISORDER OF INFANCY
INTERVIEW FORM

1. Does the infant engage in repeated regurgitation of foods, not preceded by nausea, retching, or disgust?
2. For how long has this behavior been observed?
3. Has he or she been eating normally before these episodes appeared?
4. Has he or she experienced weight loss or failure to gain expected weight for the developmental age?
5. Is this behavior associated with a physical disorder?
6. How has the caretaker been affected by the infant's periods of repeated regurgitation?
7. Are any developmental delays suspected?

RUMINATION DISORDER OF INFANCY
CASE SUMMARY - Penny, C.A., 6 months

Penny was admitted to the hospital for evaluation of failure to thrive. She was the product of a full-term, uncomplicated pregnancy, with normal labor and delivery. At birth, she weighed 6-1/2 pounds, was in good condition, and had no difficulties in the neonatal period. She was initially breastfed.

At 6 weeks, because of vomiting, her mother changed her to formula feeding. The vomiting continued in spite of numerous formula changes, and at 6 months of age she weighed only 9 pounds. Medical evaluation found no pathology other than esophagitis secondary to vomiting. Penny was observed to induce vomiting either by her hands or by tongue thrusting.

CHECKLIST

RUMINATION DISORDER OF INFANCY

Major Symptoms:

Key

-	Inattention	
-	Impulsivity	
-	Abnormal Activity Level	
-	Aggressiveness	
-	Violation of Rules	
-	Isolation/Withdrawal/Avoidance	
-	Inability to Form/Maintain Relationships	
-	Disturbances of Affect or Mood	
-	Anxiety	
-	Depression	
-	Delusions/Hallucinations	
-	Somatic Complaints	
+	Oddities of Behavior	
-	Language Impairment	
*	Impaired Cognition	

Key

+ Presence

- Absence

* Associated
  Feature

Demographic Variables:

Age of Onset: Usually between 3 and 12 months of age.
Duration: At least 1 month.

Treatment focused on directing Penny's interpersonal stimulation outward. This necessitated a 3-week hospital stay during which nursing, psychological, and occupational therapy worked intensively with Penny and her mother.

AUTHORS' COMMENTS

This case clearly illustrates the pattern of Rumination Disorder of Infancy. In such cases a complete developmental evaluation is indicated to rule out delays in other areas of the infant's functioning brought about by the lack of food retention.

ADDITIONAL READINGS
FOR EATING DISORDERS

Abraham, S., & Llewellyn-Jones, D. (1987). *Eating Disorders: The Facts.* New York: Oxford University Press.

Bicknell, J. D. (1975). *Pica: A Childhood Symptom.* London: Butterworths.

Burrows, G. D., Beumont, P., & Casper, R. C. (Eds.). (1988). *Handbook of Eating Disorders.* New York: Elsevier Science Publication Co.

Domangue, B. B., & Field, H. L. (Eds.). (1987). *Eating Disorders Throughout the Life Span.* New York: Praeger.

Mitchell, J. E. (Ed.). (1985). *Anorexia Nervosa and Bulimia: Diagnosis and Treatment.* Minneapolis: University of Minnesota Press.

Newman, P. A., & Halvorson, P. A. (1983). *Anorexia Nervosa and Bulimia: A Handbook for Counselors and Therapists.* New York: Van Nostrand Reinhold.

SLEEP DISORDERS

INTRODUCTION

During the course of parental interviews, information concerning the child's sleep patterns may be reported to the mental health professional. Common parental complaints include nightmares and sleepwalking.

The following syndromes have been selected because of their incidence and age of onset from a more comprehensive group of sleep disorders described in the *DSM-III-R*.

DREAM ANXIETY DISORDER
(NIGHTMARE DISORDER)

This newly defined category of sleep disorder is characterized by frequent sleep interruptions due to vivid dreams which are usually threatening and frightening to the child. Upon awakening, the child is oriented and alert, is able to recall the dream in detail, but becomes distressed by its content, and is usually unable to go back to sleep. Common themes of such nightmares include threats to survival, security, or self-esteem.

Nightmare episodes tend to occur during REM (rapid eye movement) sleep. Because this period of sleep inhibits body movement, the parent does not usually notice physical signs of agitation in the child.

Over half of the reported cases of Dream Anxiety Disorder occur before the age of 10, and in about 60% of the cases, the onset follows a major stressful life event. Frequency of episodes varies among individuals; it can occur three or more times per week. This disorder appears to be more prevalent in children who suffer from physical and mental health problems.

CHECKLIST

DREAM ANXIETY DISORDER
(NIGHTMARE DISORDER)

Major Symptoms:

		Key
-	Inattention	+ Presence
-	Impulsivity	- Absence
-	Abnormal Activity Level	* Associated Feature
-	Aggressiveness	
-	Violation of Rules	
-	Isolation/Withdrawal/Avoidance	
-	Inability to Form/Maintain Relationships	
-	Disturbances of Affect or Mood	
+	Anxiety	
-	Depression	
-	Delusions/Hallucinations	
-	Somatic Complaints	
-	Oddities of Behavior	
-	Language Impairment	
-	Impaired Cognition	

Demographic Variables:

Age of Onset: Before age 10.
Duration: Variable.

DREAM ANXIETY DISORDER
(NIGHTMARE DISORDER)
INTERVIEW FORM

1. Does the child exhibit repeated interruptions in sleep because of frightening dreams?
2. What is the content of these dreams?
3. Describe the child's behavior upon awakening.
4. When do the nightmares generally occur?
5. After awakening from a nightmare, can the child easily go back to sleep?
6. Is the child taking medication?
7. Has there been a recent stressful event in the child's life?
8. Does the child have a history of mental and/or physical health problems? Describe.

SLEEP TERROR DISORDER

Sleep Terror Disorder is differentiated from Dream Anxiety Disorder in that in Sleep Terror, there is no dream recall, a higher anxiety level, and a tendency for the episode to occur earlier in the night.

Abrupt awakening usually begins with a panicky scream; behaviors during the episode may include physiological symptoms such as perspiration, dilated pupils, and rapid pulse. Also present are perseverative movements, a frightened expression, increased anxiety, and an overall agitated state. These children are unable to respond to attempts at communication or comfort from others. Sleep Terror differs from seizures in that seizures may also manifest themselves during waking hours.

Sleep Terror episodes may last from 1 to 10 minutes, and occur after the children have been asleep from 30 minutes to 3-1/2 hours. There may be a vague recall of a sensation of panic upon awakening, but by morning there is no recollection of the Sleep Terror episode.

Social impairment may occur as a result of Sleep Terror episodes because of reluctance to go on overnight visits such as to camp or with friends. Accidental injury may take place during the episode.

Although recurrent Sleep Terror episodes are only experienced by 1% to 4% of children, isolated episodes appear to be more common. They seem to be related to a familial history of sleep disturbances and may be precipitated by stress, febrile illness, excessive fatigue, and/or bedtime medication.

CHECKLIST

SLEEP TERROR DISORDER

Major Symptoms:

Key

-	Inattention
-	Impulsivity
-	Abnormal Activity Level
-	Aggressiveness
-	Violation of Rules
*	Isolation/Withdrawal/Avoidance
-	Inability to Form/Maintain Relationships
-	Disturbances of Affect or Mood
+	Anxiety
-	Depression
-	Delusions/Hallucinations
-	Somatic Complaints
+	Oddities of Behavior
-	Language Impairment
-	Impaired Cognition

Key

+ Presence

- Absence

* Associated
  Feature

Demographic Variables:

Age of Onset: Between 4 and 12 years of age.
Duration: Variable.

130

SLEEP TERROR DISORDER
INTERVIEW FORM

1. For how long has the child been asleep before the onset of the episode?
2. Does the Sleep Terror episode begin with a panicky scream?
3. How long does the episode last?
4. Does the child experience any of the following during the episode: sweating, piloerection, tachycardia, rapid breathing, dilated pupils, or intense anxiety?
5. Does the child remember the episode in the morning?
6. Describe behaviors and responses to attempts at arousal.
7. Does the child suffer from seizures or CNS complications?
8. Is there a familial history of sleep disturbances?
9. Has the child recently been under stress or overly fatigued?
10. Is the child taking medication; if so, what kind and when taken?
11. Is the child reluctant to go on overnight visits?

SLEEP TERROR DISORDER
CASE SUMMARY - Jane, C.A., 4-2

Jane, a 4-year-old girl, was brought to the pediatrician because of extremely severe nightmares. For about 6 weeks she had been awakening three to four times a week screaming. This usually occurred in the late evening while the parents were still awake. Her parents would rush into her room each time and attempt to determine the reason for her upset. The child was very difficult to engage and unable to say what the trouble was. The next morning she would not recall the incident. Usually, after a few minutes with her parents, she would resume sleep. Jane had no other unpredictable episodic behaviors for the remainder of the day. There was no unusual stress or discernible significant trauma in the recent past.

Jane was completely normal upon examination. She was felt to have a simple Sleep Terror Disorder. Valium in low dosage was prescribed for 2 weeks, with gradual withdrawal from the medication after that. The episodes ceased and did not recur.

AUTHORS' COMMENTS

Jane's nightmares occurred several hours after going to sleep. She woke up screaming and was unable to be aroused by her parents during the episode. Jane could not recall the incident the next morning. Her physical manifestations during the episodes, other than her screaming, were not available. Duration of each episode was not reported.

The difference between Sleep Terror and Dream Anxiety Disorder is that the former tends to occur earlier during the night and begins with a scream. In addition, the child is unable to recall the dream and falls back asleep immediately.

SLEEPWALKING DISORDER

This disorder is characterized by walking during sleep. The episode may last from a few minutes to one-half hour. The child usually arises from bed after being asleep for at least 30 minutes to 3-1/2 hours. The episode may involve purposeful or perseverative motor movements, including dressing, opening doors, eating, or going to the bathroom. Sometimes it may only include motor movements in bed.

When sleepwalking, these children have a blank look and are unresponsive to attempts at communicating with them, awakening only through major efforts by adults. When they wake up, they may seem confused, disoriented for a few minutes, and most likely unable to recall the episode of sleepwalking.

Social impairment may occur because of reluctance to go on overnight visits such as camp or to the home of friends. Because of poor balance and motor coordination during the episode of sleepwalking, physical injury may occur.

Isolated episodes of sleepwalking have been estimated to occur in as many as 15% of all children. Chronic sleepwalking is said to account for only 1% to 6%, usually occurring between the ages of 6 and 12. Children are more prone to this disorder if there is a familial history of sleepwalking, or if they suffer from febrile illness, seizures, CNS infections, trauma, excessive fatigue, stress, or the effects of bedtime medication.

CHECKLIST

SLEEPWALKING DISORDER

Major Symptoms:

Key

-	Inattention
-	Impulsivity
-	Abnormal Activity Level
-	Aggressiveness
-	Violation of Rules
*	Isolation/Withdrawal/Avoidance
-	Inability to Form/Maintain Relationships
-	Disturbances of Affect or Mood
-	Anxiety
-	Depression
-	Delusions/Hallucinations
-	Somatic Complaints
+	Oddities of Behavior
-	Language Impairment
-	Impaired Cognition

Key

+ Presence

- Absence

* Associated
  Feature

Demographic Variables:

Age of Onset: Between 6 and 12 years of age.
Duration: Variable.

133

SLEEPWALKING DISORDER
INTERVIEW FORM

1. For how long has the child been asleep before the onset of the episode?
2. Describe behaviors and responses to attempts at arousal.
3. Does the child remember the episode?
4. When the child wakes up, is he or she confused and disoriented? If so, for how long?
5. Do sleepwalking-like behaviors occur during waking hours?
6. Is there a familial history of sleep disturbances?
7. Has the child recently been under stress or overly fatigued?
8. Is the child taking medication? If so, what kind and when is it taken?
9. Is the child reluctant to go on overnight visits?
10. Does the child suffer from seizures or CNS complications?

ADDITIONAL READINGS
FOR SLEEP DISORDERS

Ablon, S. L., & Mack, J. E. (1979). Sleep disorders. In J. Noshpitz (Ed.), *Basic Handbook of Child Psychiatry* (Vol. 2, pp. 643-660). New York: Basic Books.

Erman, M. K. (Guest Ed.). (1987). Sleep disorders. *Psychiatric Clinics of North America, 10,* 517-724.

Guilleminault, C. (Ed.). (1987). *Sleep and Its Disorders in Children.* New York: Raven Press.

IMPULSE CONTROL DISORDERS

KLEPTOMANIA

Unlike the *DSM-III*, the *DSM-III-R* requires that a motive for stealing, such as anger or vengeance, be ruled out when considering a diagnosis of Kleptomania.

Kleptomania refers to the inability to control recurrent impulses to take objects that do not belong to the individual in question, and for which he or she does not have any specific use, either personally or for financial gain. Objects taken are usually returned, presented as gifts, or hidden from sight.

The stealing event is commonly preceded by heightened tension, with pleasurable feelings of relief upon commission of the act. The stealing is not done as an act of anger or vengeance against others.

One differentiation between Kleptomania and common acts of stealing is that the individual with this disorder is financially able to acquire the given objects legally. Another important difference is that Kleptomania is usually a solitary act and one that does not involve conscious prior planning. An individual unable to control his or her impulses does not consider the consequences and ramifications of being caught. However, he or she freely expresses anxiety and worry at the possibility of being discovered and may feel depressed at his or her inability to control such impulses.

Episodes of Kleptomania do not necessarily occur with regularity; however, they can continue to manifest themselves sporadically for many years.

(Consult Checklist on page 138.)

KLEPTOMANIA
INTERVIEW FORM

1. Does the person talk about trying to resist the impulse to steal?
2. How does the person describe his or her feelings prior to and during the stealing episode?

137

CHECKLIST

KLEPTOMANIA

Major Symptoms:

Key

-	Inattention
+	Impulsivity
-	Abnormal Activity Level
-	Aggressiveness
+	Violation of Rules
-	Isolation/Withdrawal/Avoidance
-	Inability to Form/Maintain Relationships
-	Disturbances of Affect or Mood
+	Anxiety
*	Depression
-	Delusions/Hallucinations
-	Somatic Complaints
-	Oddities of Behavior
-	Language Impairment
-	Impaired Cognition

Key
+ Presence
- Absence
* Associated Feature

Demographic Variables:

Age of Onset: Childhood.
Duration: Variable.

3. Is the person's motivation for stealing, anger or need for revenge?
4. Does the person perceive a use or need for the stolen object?
5. Has the person been diagnosed as having a Conduct Disorder?
6. Is the person financially able to purchase the object in question?
7. Does the person report prior planning of the act?
8. Does the person steal alone or as part of a group?
9. What does the person do once the object is in his or her possession?
10. Is the person able to think clearly about the consequences of his or her actions when not engaged in stealing?
11. Is the person able to express remorse or fear of being caught at times other than when he or she is stealing?

PYROMANIA

Unlike the *DSM-III*, the *DSM-III-R* requires that a motive for committing the fire-setting, such as anger or vengeance, be ruled out when considering a diagnosis of Pyromania.

Pyromania refers to the inability to resist a specific impulse to set fires. Fascination with fire may be exhibited by setting false alarms, by frequent visits to local fire stations, and by eager participation in watching fires, especially those set by the individual himself or herself.

The individual feels increased tension preceding the fire-setting, with release and extreme gratification at seeing the results of the act. Often these individuals take elaborate measures to plan and execute the burning; however, because of their intense involvement in the act and their poor impulse control, they are careless at protecting themselves from being discovered, leaving behind obvious clues.

In spite of possible dangerous consequences, these individuals appear oblivious to the damage and destruction their behavior causes. In this disorder, however, fire-setting is not done primarily to express anger or vengeance towards others, for monetary gain, or as part of delusionary or hallucinatory thinking.

Below-average IQ, sexual arousal during fire-setting, chronic resentment against authority, and low frustration tolerance are features often associated with this disorder.

(Consult Checklist on page 141.)

PYROMANIA
INTERVIEW FORM

1. How often has the individual been involved in fire-setting behavior?
2. How does the individual describe his or her feelings prior to the fire-setting and during its commission?
3. Does the individual seem unusually interested in fire-fighting equipment, visiting fire houses, and the like?
4. What is the individual's motivation for setting fires?
5. Has the individual been caught setting off fire alarms?
6. Is the individual concerned about the consequences of setting fires, such as damage to property, or endangering the life of others?
7. Is the individual resistive to authority?
8. How does the individual cope with everyday frustrating situations?

PYROMANIA
CASE SUMMARY - John, C.A., 6-3

Psychiatric Summary: This 6-year-old boy was hospitalized after he set fire to a scrap basket in the bathroom of his house. He was brought in by his mother and the social worker from the Department of Children and Youth Services (DCYS), both of whom requested hospitalization to provide relief from the tension between parent and child and to establish therapeutic counseling.

This was not the first time John had set fires. He once burned his mother's hair with a lighter, set the apartment curtains on fire, "vacuumed" the rug with a heated iron, and pulled the electric burner out of the stove.

On examination, he was a normal boy who was pleasant, verbal, and cooperative although obviously anxious. He was relieved to be in a safe environment. He and his

CHECKLIST

PYROMANIA

Major Symptoms:

Key

-	Inattention
+	Impulsivity
-	Abnormal Activity Level
+	Aggressiveness
+	Violation of Rules
-	Isolation/Withdrawal/Avoidance
-	Inability to Form/Maintain Relationships
-	Disturbances of Affect or Mood
+	Anxiety
-	Depression
-	Delusions/Hallucinations
-	Somatic Complaints
-	Oddities of Behavior
-	Language Impairment
-	Impaired Cognition

Key

+ Presence

- Absence

* Associated
  Feature

Demographic Variables:

Age of Onset: Childhood.
Duration: Variable.

mother readily established therapeutic relationships with the social worker and therapists. After 10 days of intensive intervention, John was discharged to continue with outpatient individual and family therapy with DCYS supervision.

John had a second hospitalization 9 months later, when he was again "out of control" and his mother pleaded for help as she felt she was likely to abuse him. Six months later he was admitted to an inpatient psychiatric hospital for children.

AUTHORS' COMMENTS

John presents a continuous pattern of fire-setting, primarily at home. The Clinical Summary does not provide information about John's feelings towards his mother, or his awareness of the consequences of his actions. Despite the limited information provided, a diagnosis of Pyromania seems appropriate in view of John's repeated fire-setting behaviors.

ADDITIONAL READINGS FOR
IMPULSE CONTROL DISORDERS

Gaynor, J., & Hatcher, C. (1987). *The Psychology of Child Firesetting: Detection and Intervention.* New York: Brunner-Mazel.

Kuhnley, E. J., Hendren, R., & Quinlan, D. (1982). Firesetting by children. *Journal of the American Academy of Child Psychiatry, 21,* 560-563.

Monroe, R. R. (1970). *Episodic Behavioral Disorders: A Psychodynamic and Neurophysiologic Analysis.* Cambridge: Harvard University Press.

ELIMINATION DISORDERS

INTRODUCTION

These disorders include Functional Enuresis and Functional Encopresis. They are included in this book because of their impact on a child's self-image and social functioning. Children with these disorders suffer embarrassment, low self-esteem, and negative reactions such as anger, punishment, and rejection from caretakers. Impairment in social functioning may be characterized by avoidance of overnight activities, ostracism, and teasing by peers.

FUNCTIONAL ENURESIS

This disorder involves the inability to control the voiding of urine, at night and/or during the day, after an age where such control would be expected. For such a diagnosis to be made, a physical cause such as diabetes, urinary tract infection, or seizure disorder must be ruled out. Furthermore, to obtain a diagnosis of Functional Enuresis, the voiding must occur two or more times per month for a child between the ages of 5 and 6, and one or more times per month for older children.

The *DSM-III-R* differentiates between primary and secondary Enuresis. In the first type, children have not yet achieved or maintained continence for at least a year. In the second type, children have been continent for more than a year before the onset of Enuresis. Children cannot be diagnosed as having primary Enuresis before age 5; secondary Enuresis is usually identified from ages 5 to 8.

Either type of Enuresis can be diurnal, nocturnal, or both. Diurnal Enuresis refers to the voiding of urine during waking hours. In nocturnal Enuresis, voiding occurs during sleep with no recollection by the child of having had an "accident."

This disorder is relatively common and may be precipitated by stressful events, such as birth of a sibling, entering school, or changing neighborhoods.

CHECKLIST

FUNCTIONAL ENURESIS

Major Symptoms:

-	Inattention
-	Impulsivity
-	Abnormal Activity Level
-	Aggressiveness
-	Violation of Rules
*	Isolation/Withdrawal/Avoidance
*	Inability to Form/Maintain Relationships
-	Disturbances of Affect or Mood
-	Anxiety
-	Depression
-	Delusions/Hallucinations
-	Somatic Complaints
-	Oddities of Behavior
-	Language Impairment
-	Impaired Cognition

Key

+ Presence

- Absence

* Associated Feature

Demographic Variables:

Age of Onset: By age 5.
Duration: Two or more times per month for children between ages 5 and 6, and one or more times for older children.

146

FUNCTIONAL ENURESIS
INTERVIEW FORM

1. Does the child show repeated voiding of urine during waking or sleeping times, regardless of whether it is intentional or not?
2. When are these episodes most prevalent?
3. How often do these occur?
4. Has a recent medical examination ruled out physical causes for the enuresis?
5. Was toilet training achieved prior to the onset of enuresis? If yes, at what age?
6. What are the chronological and mental ages of the child?
7. Does the child feel embarrassed or does he or she avoid social situations as a result of the enuresis?
8. Has the child recently been under unusual stress, such as the birth of a sibling, hospitalization, or entering school?
9. What management techniques have been attempted by the caretakers to control the child's voiding?

FUNCTIONAL ENURESIS
CASE SUMMARY - Harold, C.A., 8-2

Harold, an 8-year-old boy, was brought to the psychologist because his continued nightly bedwetting prevented him from sleeping at friends' homes or participating in overnight camping with the Cub Scouts. He and his family sought help, as their attempts at managing his enuresis - using after-dinner deprivation of liquids and awakening him in the late evening - did not work. The boy and his mother were having increasingly hostile interchanges over the wetting situation. He was dry during the daytime.

The medical history was not significant. Recent physical examination ruled out urinary tract infection and kidney dysfunction. Overall, Harold was developing normally and had been toilet trained easily by age 3. The onset of bedwetting had occurred 2 years before, coinciding with the birth of a sibling.

Harold was started on a conditioning system using a bell to awaken him when wetting began. He was also given the responsibility to change his pajamas and bedding. A reward system using a chart was initiated. Gradual improvement was noted as soon as 1 week. Three months were required before he felt secure enough to go away from home for an overnight trip. There was no relapse when the alarm system was discontinued.

AUTHORS' COMMENTS

Harold shows repeated inability to control urination during the nighttime hours. Referral was made because of the social implications of his voiding behaviors at home and away from home. A medical examination ruled out physical reasons for Harold's incontinence.

Toilet training was achieved at the expected developmental age; thus, a diagnosis of nocturnal Functional Enuresis, secondary type, was made.

FUNCTIONAL ENCOPRESIS

This disorder involves involuntary or in rare cases intentional bowel movements, not due to the presence of a physical condition, and discharged in places other than the toilet. Constipation may be frequent, and may occur because the child experiences anxiety about defecating in a specific place, or refuses to defecate because of an overall pattern of oppositional behaviors. For such diagnosis to be made, children must be at least 4 years old, and episodes of Encopresis must occur at least once per month for a period of at least 6 months.

The *DSM-III-R* differentiates between primary and secondary Encopresis. In the first type, the child has not yet achieved or been able to maintain fecal continence for at least 1 year. In the second type, the child has been continent for at least 1 year before the onset of Encopresis. The earliest that a diagnosis of primary Functional Encopresis can be made is age 4, while secondary Functional Encopresis may be diagnosed from ages 4 to 8.

This disorder may be precipitated by stressful events such as birth of a sibling or entering school. Intentional release of feces may be associated with antisocial behavior or other clinical syndromes. According to the *DSM-III-R*, Functional Enuresis is present in about 25% of children who have also been diagnosed as having Functional Encopresis.

The effects of this disorder on self-esteem and overall social functioning parallel those found in the disorder of Functional Enuresis.

CHECKLIST

FUNCTIONAL ENCOPRESIS

Major Symptoms:

Key

-	Inattention
-	Impulsivity
-	Abnormal Activity Level
*	Aggressiveness
*	Violation of Rules
*	Isolation/Withdrawal/Avoidance
*	Inability to Form/Maintain Relationships
-	Disturbances of Affect or Mood
*	Anxiety
-	Depression
-	Delusions/Hallucinations
-	Somatic Complaints
+	Oddities of Behavior
-	Language Impairment
-	Impaired Cognition

Key:
+ Presence
- Absence
* Associated Feature

Demographic Variables:

Age of Onset: By age 4.
Duration: At least one event per month for at least 6 months.

FUNCTIONAL ENCOPRESIS
INTERVIEW FORM

1. Does the child defecate in inappropriate places?
2. How often does this occur?
3. What are the child's chronological and mental ages?
4. Has a recent medical examination ruled out physical causes for the Encopresis?
5. Was toilet training of bowel movements achieved prior to the onset of Encopresis? If yes, at what age?
6. Does the child feel embarrassed or does he or she avoid social situations as a result of Encopresis?
7. Has the child recently been under unusual stress, such as birth of a sibling, hospitalization, or entering school?
8. Does the child become anxious when expected to defecate in a specific place?
9. Is the child's defecation in inappropriate places, a deliberate behavior?
10. Does the child show any oppositional or antisocial behaviors such as excessive aggressiveness, temper tantrums, asociality, or destruction of property?
11. Does the child suffer from constipation?
12. What management techniques have been attempted by the caretakers to deal with the child's Encopresis?

FUNCTIONAL ENCOPRESIS
CASE SUMMARY - Jason, C.A., 7-9

Jason, a 7-1/2-year-old boy, was admitted to the hospital for treatment of Encopresis as attempted outpatient management had failed. His family reported that he had never been successfully bowel trained.

Toilet training was begun shortly before the birth of a younger sibling when Jason was 2 years old. By age 4, he was continent of urine but not of stool. He normally soiled twice a day, before and after school. A gastroenterologist was consulted and the appropriate studies were done to rule out an organic cause.

When Jason was 6 years old, he was referred to a behavioral clinic. He was started on the usual regimen of cleansing enemas, stool softener, and scheduled times on the toilet, with rewards for clean pants, bowel movements in the toilet, and complying with medication. He did well initially, using a star chart and trading in stars for material rewards. After acquiring cable TV as a reward, he quit taking the medication and complying with the contract. Soiling resumed.

Jason was then begun on cleansing enemas, followed by stool softeners and a regular toileting schedule. A contract was agreed upon in which primary responsibility was placed on Jason. Bowel continence was promptly achieved.

A psychological evaluation was obtained because of the prolonged course of the disorder with prior medical management. He was found to be in the Superior range of measured intelligence. The personality assessment indicated withdrawal as his primary strategy. Jason indicated awareness of his needs but hesitation to seek fulfillment through others. He perceived closeness to others as associated with loss, and thus avoided involvement.

Because of these findings and observations of his tendency to withdraw while hospitalized, recommendations were made for individual and family psychotherapy. He was discharged after 2 weeks of combined medical and psychological management. On follow-up, Jason continued to be continent 1 year later.

AUTHORS' COMMENTS

Jason presents a long-term pattern of fecal incontinence which has been continuous since an early age, with no success in bowel training when such milestones are usually acquired.

A medical examination ruled out physical causes for his incontinence. Because defecation was initially related to school (before and after), this was the apparent stressor. His tendency to avoid interaction with others may be considered a more recent social stressor.

A diagnosis of Primary Functional Encopresis was made.

ADDITIONAL READINGS
FOR ELIMINATION DISORDERS

Butler, R. J. (1987). *Nocturnal Enuresis: Psychological Perspectives.* Bristol: Wright.

Schafer, C. E. (1979). *Childhood Encopresis and Enuresis: Causes and Therapy.* New York: Van Nostrand Reinhold.

TIC
DISORDERS

INTRODUCTION

This group of disorders was formerly known as Stereotyped Movement Disorders in the *DSM-III*. Major changes in the *DSM-III-R* include the consideration of vocal as well as motor tics, the differentiation between simple and complex tics, and some differences in the duration and frequency of their manifestation.

Tic Disorders are characterized by abnormalities in gross motor movement. Tourette's Disorder, Transient Tic Disorder, and Chronic Motor or Vocal Tic Disorder all involve tics. Tics are defined as involuntary, rapid production of noises, words, or muscle movements. They may be controlled for a certain period of time despite their compelling nature.

Both motor and vocal tics may be classified as simple or complex. Simple motor tics include eye blinking, neck jerking, shoulder shrugging, and facial grimacing. Simple vocal tics may include coughing, throat clearing, grunting, sniffing, snorting, and barking. Complex motor tics include facial gestures, grooming behaviors, hitting or biting oneself, jumping, touching, stamping, smelling an object, or mimicking someone else. Complex vocal tics include repetition of words or phrases out of context, use of socially unacceptable words, echolalia, and repeating oneself.

Self-consciousness, embarrassment, and social alienation are common. Impairment in daily activities, such as reading and writing, may occur as a result of tics. Tics, in general, tend to decrease during nonanxious, concentrated activities, and during sleep, while generally increasing during periods of stress and tension.

TOURETTE'S DISORDER

This disorder involves a multiple tic condition. It is characterized by muscle tics, particularly of the head, torso, and limbs, accompanied by vocal tics. These occur several times a day, nearly every day, or intermittently, and should be present for at least 1 year prior to a diagnosis. The number and combination of simple and complex tics changes over time. Vocal tics range from sounds to grunts, barks, coughs, and words. In up to one-third of the cases, utterances of obscenities are common. All of these symptoms tend to appear during stressful situations, but are lessened during nonanxious events or absorption in an activity, and are not present during sleep.

Other symptoms may involve imitative physical movements, vocalizations, obsessive/compulsive behaviors or thoughts, ritualistic behaviors, and a tendency to repeat words or phrases. In over 50% of these cases there is a secondary diagnosis of Attention Deficit Hyperactivity Disorder and/or Learning Disabilities. The most common learning problem is handwriting. Children with this disorder are usually described as irritable, with low frustration tolerance and attentional problems. They tend to show slower overall maturational processes, yet they often have an average IQ.

Initially this disorder may manifest itself with a solitary tic and advance to the multiple range of behaviors described above. In other cases, multiple symptoms are present from the onset in any combination and are usually aggravated during adolescence.

The social and emotional consequences of this disorder may range from discomfort in social situations to more serious depressive and suicidal tendencies. Other complications may include physical injuries as a result of the complex motor tics.

(Consult Checklist on page 157.)

TOURETTE'S DISORDER
INTERVIEW FORM

1. Does the child exhibit physical tics? Describe.
2. Does the child vocalize strange noises such as grunts, yelps, clicks, or barks?
3. How often do tics occur?
4. For how long has the child been exhibiting these involuntary behaviors?
5. At what age were the symptoms first observed?

CHECKLIST

TOURETTE'S DISORDER

Major Symptoms:

Key

*	Inattention
*	Impulsivity
*	Abnormal Activity Level
-	Aggressiveness
-	Violation of Rules
*	Isolation/Withdrawal/Avoidance
*	Inability to Form/Maintain Relationships
-	Disturbances of Affect or Mood
*	Anxiety
*	Depression
-	Delusions/Hallucinations
-	Somatic Complaints
+	Oddities of Behavior
-	Language Impairment
-	Impaired Cognition

Key
+ Presence
- Absence
* Associated Feature

Demographic Variables:

Age of Onset: Median age is 7 years; can occur between 1 and 14 years.
Duration: More than 1 year.

6. Has a medical examination shown neurological abnormalities?
7. Do the symptoms occur exclusively during substance intoxication?
8. Does the child vocalize obscenities without provocation?
9. Is the child able to voluntarily control the physical and vocal tics? For how long?
10. Does the child imitate the movements or utterances of others?
11. Does he or she exhibit obsessive/compulsive behaviors such as constant self-doubt, need to touch things, or need to perform complex physical movements?
12. Describe the degree of social/academic impairment being experienced by the child.

TOURETTE'S DISORDER
CASE SUMMARY - Bob, C.A., 13-1

Referral Information: Bob's Social Studies teacher referred him for evaluation because she had observed nervous mannerisms, such as facial tics and guttural sounds, and felt that his achievement level was significantly low. Bob had previously been evaluated. At that time, his cognitive functioning was found to be in the Average range, although he showed signs of excessive emotionality.

Behavioral Observations: Bob was observed in the Social Studies class; he tossed his head, squinted, and uttered monosyllabic sounds in what appeared to be an involuntary rhythmic pattern. In the evaluative situation, Bob was attentive and cooperative. A combination of tic-like phenomena began midway through the first subtest, consisting of eye blinking, grimacing, and short "hup, hup" sounds that he attempted to cover up by saying "Oh, gosh." This continued through the remainder of testing. At the second session he was again able to control the distracting behaviors for about 15 minutes, but this time, his short "barked" words seemed to be coprolalic in nature.

Test Interpretations: On the WISC-R, Bob earned Verbal, Performance, and Full Scale scores in the Average range of cognitive ability. Bob's reproductions of the Bender Gestalt were without error. He worked carefully and slowly, making several auto-critical comments. There was an obsessive/compulsive flavor to his drawings.

Additional projective testing suggested that Bob's feelings of inadequacy and isolation generate a sense of anger, depression, and frustration. His main defenses appear to be regression and fantasy.

Recommendation: It is strongly recommended that Bob's parents schedule him for a thorough neurological examination to confirm or rule out what may be a physical disorder for which there could be appropriate medication. There are indications that Bob may be a youngster of bright average potential, but the cluster of symptoms he manifests may be interfering with his expected social and academic development.

Neurologist's Report to School: I have been following Bob for a period of 8 months and have him on Haldol because of a tic disorder. All indications are that he has Tourette's Disorder.

AUTHORS' COMMENTS

Bob presents the typical symptoms of Tourette's Disorder: facial tics, guttural sounds, vocalization of obscenities, as well as attempts at controlling such behaviors. Associated features described in Bob's protocol included obsessive/compulsive behaviors, low self-esteem, anxiety, and depression. Bob's multiple tics were more evident during times of particular stress, especially during formal testing.

Impairment in academic performance has been noted. The extent of his social impairment is not clear from the report. There is no indication as to the duration, frequency, and intensity of the tic behaviors.

CHRONIC MOTOR OR
VOCAL TIC DISORDER

This disorder is characterized by either motor or vocal tics, but not both. Their severity and consequent functional impairment is less significant than in Tourette's Disorder.

CHECKLIST

CHRONIC MOTOR OR
VOCAL TIC DISORDER

Major Symptoms:

Key

-	Inattention
*	Impulsivity
*	Abnormal Activity Level
-	Aggressiveness
-	Violation of Rules
*	Isolation/Withdrawal/Avoidance
*	Inability to Form/Maintain Relationships
-	Disturbances of Affect or Mood
*	Anxiety
-	Depression
-	Delusions/Hallucinations
-	Somatic Complaints
+	Oddities of Behavior
-	Language Impairment
-	Impaired Cognition

Key:
+ Presence
- Absence
* Associated Feature

Demographic Variables:

Age of Onset: Before age 21.
Duration: At least 1 year.

160

CHRONIC MOTOR OR
VOCAL TIC DISORDER
INTERVIEW FORM

1. Describe the type of tics observed in the person.
2. How often do these tics occur?
3. How long have these tics been evident?
4. Do the tics occur exclusively during substance abuse?
5. Has there been a diagnosis of CNS disease, such as a history of encephalitis?
6. Is the person avoiding others as a result of embarrassment?
7. Do the tics interfere with the person's ability to function in school and/or on a job?

CHRONIC MOTOR OR
VOCAL TIC DISORDER
CASE SUMMARY - Mike, C.A., 9-0

Mike is a 9-year-old boy who was diagnosed at age 6 with Attention Deficit Disorder. Ritalin was prescribed, as well as individual and family therapy. After 2 years on Ritalin, Mike began making sniffing sounds and whistling in the classroom. The teacher called these behaviors to his mother's attention and they were reported to the prescribing physician. Ritalin was stopped; Mike's academic performance and impulse control promptly deteriorated.

Mike was hospitalized to treat both the tics and the ADD, and was started on a prescription of Clonidine. His activity level has been significantly reduced, with no evidence of tics. Mike has been able to return to his classroom.

AUTHORS' COMMENTS

This case illustrates the possible side effects of some medications. In Mike's case, Ritalin, a common drug prescribed for Attention Deficit Disorder, may have contributed to the onset of Vocal Tics. These subsided once the medication was changed.

161

TRANSIENT TIC DISORDER

This disorder involves repetitive, rapid motor movements, which may be voluntarily controlled for some period of time. Symptoms include simple, single tics which usually subside within a year. Most common transient tics are facial tics such as eye blinking; however, the entire torso, head, or limbs may be involved simultaneously or in isolation. At times, these tics may be accompanied by vocal noises.

The severity and frequency of tics varies; they generally seem to be triggered by stressful episodes and usually subside during sleep.

(Consult Checklist on page 163.)

TRANSIENT TIC DISORDER
INTERVIEW FORM

1. Does the child exhibit recurrent motor or vocal tics?
2. How often and for how long do these tics occur?
3. Has the person been diagnosed as having Tourette's Disorder or Chronic Motor or Vocal Tic Disorder?
4. At what age were these tics first noticed?
5. Do the tics occur exclusively during substance abuse?
6. Is the person avoiding others as a result of embarrassment?
7. Do the tics interfere with the person's ability to function in school and/or on the job?
8. Do these tics regularly appear in anticipation of, or during periods of stress in the person's life?

ADDITIONAL READINGS
FOR TIC DISORDERS

Cohen, D. J., Bruun, R., & Leckman, J. (Eds.). (1988). *Tourette's Syndrome and Tic Disorders: Clinical Understanding and Treatment.* New York: John Wiley.
Lees, A. J. (1985). *Tics and Related Disorders.* New York: Churchill Livingstone.

CHECKLIST

TRANSIENT TIC DISORDER

Major Symptoms:

Key

	Major Symptoms	Key
-	Inattention	+ Presence
*	Impulsivity	- Absence
*	Abnormal Activity Level	* Associated Feature
-	Aggressiveness	
-	Violation of Rules	
*	Isolation/Withdrawal/Avoidance	
*	Inability to Form/Maintain Relationships	
-	Disturbances of Affect or Mood	
*	Anxiety	
-	Depression	
-	Delusions/Hallucinations	
-	Somatic Complaints	
+	Oddities of Behavior	
-	Language Impairment	
-	Impaired Cognition	

Demographic Variables:

Age of Onset: Childhood or early adolescence; as early as 2 years of age, before 21 years of age.
Duration: At least 2 weeks, no more than 12 consecutive months.

SUMMARY CHECKLIST OF MAJOR SYMPTOMS

GLOSSARY OF MAJOR SYMPTOMS

INDEX

SUMMARY CHECKLIST OF MAJOR SYMPTOMS

167

KEY
+ Presence
− Absence
* Associated Feature

IMPAIRED COGNITION	LANGUAGE IMPAIRMENT	ODDITIES OF BEHAVIOR	SOMATIC COMPLAINTS	DELUSIONS/HALLUCINATIONS	DEPRESSION	ANXIETY	DISTURBANCES OF AFFECT OR MOOD	INABILITY TO FORM/MAINTAIN RELATIONSHIPS	ISOLATION/WITHDRAWAL/AVOIDANCE	VIOLATION OF RULES	AGGRESSIVENESS	ABNORMAL ACTIVITY LEVEL	IMPULSIVITY	INATTENTION	DISORDERS
−	−	−	−	−	−	−	−	*	−	−	−	+	+	+	ATTENTION DEFICIT HYPERACTIVITY DISORDER
*	−	−	−	−	*	*	−	+	+	+	+	−	−	*	CONDUCT DISORDER, SOLITARY AGGRESSIVE TYPE
*	−	−	−	−	*	*	−	−	−	+	+	−	−	*	CONDUCT DISORDER, GROUP TYPE
−	−	−	−	−	−	−	−	*	−	+	+	−	−	−	OPPOSITIONAL DEFIANT DISORDER
−	*	−	−	−	−	+	−	+	+	−	−	−	−	−	AVOIDANT DISORDER OF CHILDHOOD OR ADOLESCENCE
−	−	−	*	−	*	+	−	*	+	−	−	−	−	−	SOCIAL PHOBIA
−	−	*	+	−	−	+	−	*	*	−	−	−	−	−	OVERANXIOUS DISORDER
−	−	−	+	−	*	+	−	+	+	−	*	−	−	−	SEPARATION ANXIETY DISORDER
−	−	−	*	*	*	+	*	*	+	−	*	*	*	*	POST-TRAUMATIC STRESS DISORDER
−	−	−	−	−	+	−	+	*	−	−	−	−	−	*	ADJUSTMENT DISORDER WITH DEPRESSED MOOD
−	−	−	−	−	−	+	+	*	−	−	−	−	−	*	ADJUSTMENT DISORDER WITH ANXIOUS MOOD
−	−	−	−	−	−	−	−	*	−	+	*	−	*	*	ADJUSTMENT DISORDER WITH DISTURBANCE OF CONDUCT
−	−	−	−	−	−	−	−	*	+	−	−	−	−	*	ADJUSTMENT DISORDER WITH WITHDRAWAL

Clinical Evaluations of School-Aged Children

KEY

- **+** Presence
- **−** Absence
- ***** Associated Feature

IMPAIRED COGNITION	LANGUAGE IMPAIRMENT	ODDITIES OF BEHAVIOR	SOMATIC COMPLAINTS	DELUSIONS/HALLUCINATIONS	DEPRESSION	ANXIETY	DISTURBANCES OF AFFECT OR MOOD	INABILITY TO FORM/MAINTAIN RELATIONSHIPS	ISOLATION/WITHDRAWAL/AVOIDANCE	VIOLATION OF RULES	AGGRESSIVENESS	ABNORMAL ACTIVITY LEVEL	IMPULSIVITY	INATTENTION	MAJOR SYMPTOMS / DISORDERS
−	−	−	+	−	−	*	−	*	−	−	−	−	−	*	ADJUSTMENT DISORDER WITH PHYSICAL COMPLAINTS
−	−	−	−	−	*	*	*	−	−	−	−	−	−	*	ADJUSTMENT DISORDER WITH WORK OR ACADEMIC INHIBITION
−	−	−	−	−	*	*	+	*	−	−	−	−	−	*	ADJUSTMENT DISORDER WITH MIXED EMOTIONAL FEATURES
−	−	−	−	−	*	*	+	*	−	+	*	−	*	*	ADJUSTMENT DISORDER WITH MIXED DISTURBANCE OF EMOTIONS AND CONDUCT
+	+	+	−	−	−	−	+	+	−	−	−	*	*	*	AUTISTIC DISORDER
+	+	+	−	+	*	*	+	+	+	−	−	+	−	−	SCHIZOPHRENIA
−	−	−	*	−	+	*	+	*	*	−	*	*	−	*	MAJOR DEPRESSIVE EPISODE/DYSTHYMIA
−	*	+	−	−	*	*	−	+	+	−	*	−	−	−	ELECTIVE MUTISM
−	−	+	−	−	*	*	−	*	*	−	−	−	−	−	GENDER IDENTITY DISORDER OF CHILDHOOD
−	−	−	−	−	+	+	*	+	−	−	−	−	−	−	IDENTITY DISORDER
−	*	−	+	−	−	−	−	+	+	−	−	+	−	+	REACTIVE ATTACHMENT DISORDER OF INFANCY AND EARLY CHILDHOOD
−	−	+	+	−	−	−	−	−	*	−	−	−	−	−	ANOREXIA NERVOSA

168

Clinical Evaluations of School-Aged Children

KEY
- **+** Presence
- **−** Absence
- ***** Associated Feature

IMPAIRED COGNITION	LANGUAGE IMPAIRMENT	ODDITIES OF BEHAVIOR	SOMATIC COMPLAINTS	DELUSIONS/HALLUCINATIONS	DEPRESSION	ANXIETY	DISTURBANCES OF AFFECT OR MOOD	INABILITY TO FORM/MAINTAIN RELATIONSHIPS	ISOLATION/WITHDRAWAL/AVOIDANCE	VIOLATION OF RULES	AGGRESSIVENESS	ABNORMAL ACTIVITY LEVEL	IMPULSIVITY	INATTENTION	MAJOR SYMPTOMS / DISORDERS
−	−	+	*	−	*	*	*	−	−	−	−	−	−	−	BULIMIA NERVOSA
*	−	+	−	−	−	−	−	−	−	−	−	−	−	−	PICA
*	−	+	−	−	−	−	−	−	−	−	−	−	−	−	RUMINATION DISORDER OF INFANCY
−	−	−	−	−	−	+	−	−	−	−	−	−	−	−	DREAM ANXIETY DISORDER (NIGHTMARE DISORDER)
−	−	+	−	−	−	+	−	−	*	−	−	−	−	−	SLEEP TERROR DISORDER
−	−	+	−	−	−	−	−	−	*	−	−	−	−	−	SLEEPWALKING DISORDER
−	−	−	−	−	*	+	−	−	−	+	−	−	+	−	KLEPTOMANIA
−	−	−	−	−	−	+	−	−	−	+	+	−	+	−	PYROMANIA
−	−	−	−	−	−	−	−	*	*	−	−	−	−	−	FUNCTIONAL ENURESIS
−	−	+	−	−	−	*	−	*	*	*	*	−	−	−	FUNCTIONAL ENCOPRESIS
−	−	+	−	−	*	*	−	*	*	−	−	*	*	*	TOURETTE'S DISORDER
−	−	+	−	−	−	*	−	*	*	−	−	*	*	−	CHRONIC MOTOR OR VOCAL TIC DISORDER
−	−	+	−	−	−	*	−	*	*	−	−	*	*	−	TRANSIENT TIC DISORDER

GLOSSARY OF MAJOR SYMPTOMS

Abnormal Activity Level: Hyperactivity or hypoactivity going beyond an expected norm.

Affect: An observable manifestation of an emotion. Affect may be recognized by the tone of voice, physical expression, body language, and altered behavioral responses.

Aggressiveness: Unprovoked verbal and/or physical attacks on people and/or property.

Anxiety: Generally defined as an advanced response to threat not necessarily objectively apparent. It distinguishes itself from fear in that the latter is more likely to concern itself with known and external sources of danger. Despite their differing sources, fear and anxiety manifest themselves in a similar manner, involving autonomic hyperactivity, tension, apprehension, and a state of tense alertness.

Delusions: A firmly and consistently held affirmation of a belief which is not supported by reality or by generally accepted perceptions, or which is held in spite of objective evidence. The delusional belief is divergent from the cultural norms of the individual holding it.

Depression: Marked by sadness, inactivity, feelings of dejection, and self-deprecation.

171

Hallucinations: A perception attributed to the senses, which is in fact not derived from them. It may be differentiated from illusions by the fact that the latter are misinterpretations or distortions of external stimuli.

Impaired Cognition: May include loosening of associations, incoherence, poverty of content of speech, neologisms, perseveration, blocking, or below-average IQ.

Impulsivity: A spontaneous inclination to perform an unpremeditated action. The action usually has a sudden, forceful, compelling quality and is taken without consideration for the consequences.

Inability to Form/Maintain Relationships: Incapacity to form or maintain relationships, or social avoidance of the individual by others as a result of his or her behaviors.

Inattention: The inability to maintain concentration on an object, task, or activity. The extent of deviation from such would be a measure of distractibility and inadequate attention.

Isolation/Withdrawal/Avoidance: Failure to approach others or situations because of fear, inexperience, lack of confidence, absorption in solitary activities, or social discomfort. Also may include intentional refusal to speak.

Language Impairment: Failure to reach expected language milestones, speech impediment, echolalia, or unintelligibility.

Mood: A sustained emotion capable of affecting an individual's perceptions and responses. Common manifestations of mood include euphoria, irritability, anxiety, depression, annoyance, and anger.

Oddities of Behavior: Includes behaviors of such unusual quality that they bring attention to the individual. May include hair pulling, rocking or other rhythmic movements; motor tics; food hoarding; sleepwalking; or eating nonfood substances. May also involve cross-dressing.

Somatic Complaints: Complaints of a physical nature, such as nausea, vomiting, headaches, tachycardia, and so on, for which no physical basis can be established.

Violation of Rules: Chronic violations of a variety of important rules that are reasonable and age-appropriate for the individual at home and/or school, such as truancy, stealing, substance abuse, or precocious sexual activity.

▮ INDEX

cognitive impairment
    in Autistic Disorder, 69
    in Pica, 118
    in Schizophrenia, 80-81
Conduct Disorders, 3-4, 8-18, 51
    Group Type, 9-11, 15-17
    Solitary Aggressive Type, 9, 13-15
    Undifferentiated Type, 9-10

D

delusions
    in Pervasive Developmental Disorders, 67
    in Schizophrenia, 79-80, 82
dependent behavior, 25, 37, 81, 92
depression
    in Adjustment Disorders, 52-53
    in Bulimia Nervosa, 115
    in Conduct Disorders, 9
    in Identity Disorder, 100
    in Kleptomania, 137
    in Major Depressive Episode/Dysthymia, 86-88
    in Post-Traumatic Stress Disorder, 42
    in Separation Anxiety Disorder, 37
    in Tourette's Disorder, 156
Dream Anxiety Disorder (Nightmare Disorder), 127-129
Dysthymia, 87-91

E

echolalia, 68, 155
Elective Mutism, 91-95

F

failure to thrive, 105
fears
    in Anorexia Nervosa, 111
    in Autistic Disorder, 69
    in Bulimia Nervosa, 115
    in Dream Anxiety Disorder, 127
    in Major Depressive Episode/Dysthymia, 87
    in Separation Anxiety Disorder, 37
    in Sleep Terror Disorder, 129
    in Social Phobia, 29

fire-setting, 9, 139-140
Functional Encopresis, 145, 148-151
Functional Enuresis, 145-148

G

Gender Identity Disorder of Childhood, 95-100

H

hallucinations
    in Pervasive Developmental Disorders, 67
    in Schizophrenia, 80, 82
hygiene problems, 81, 87
hyperactivity (*see also* abnormal activity level)
    in Attention Deficit Hyperactivity Disorder, 3-4

I

Identity Disorder, 100-105
illegal substance use
    in Bulimia Nervosa, 115
    in Conduct Disorders, 9
    in Major Depressive Episode/Dysthymia, 87
    in Oppositional Defiant Disorder, 18
    in Social Phobia, 30
impulsivity
    in Attention Deficit Hyperactivity Disorder, 3-4
    in Kleptomania, 137
    in Post-Traumatic Stress Disorder, 42
    in Pyromania, 139
    in Tic Disorders, 155
inattention
    in Attention Deficit Hyperactivity Disorder, 3-4
    in Conduct Disorders, 9
    in Major Depressive Episode/Dysthymia, 87-88
    in Post-Traumatic Stress Disorder, 42
    in Tourette's Disorder, 156
interpersonal relationships
    in Adjustment Disorders, 52
    in Attention Deficit Hyperactivity Disorder, 4